Italian Cookbook for everyday use.

Everyday cookbook series., Volume 2

Maleb Braine

Published by Maleb Braine, 2022.

While every precaution has been taken in the preparation of this book, the publisher assumes no responsibility for errors or omissions, or for damages resulting from the use of the information contained herein.

ITALIAN COOKBOOK FOR EVERYDAY USE.

First edition. September 27, 2022.

Copyright © 2022 Maleb Braine.

ISBN: 978-1915666048

Written by Maleb Braine.

Also by Maleb Braine

Everyday cookbook series.
French cookbook for everyday use.
Italian Cookbook for everyday use.
Bread baking cookbook you need every day
A baking cookbook you need Every Day

Book Description

If you have ever wondered how you can improve both your skills in the kitchen as well as your life in general, then you will find that mastering Italian cooking is the way to go.

The ideal ingredients to any happy home are the love for life and for good food! Italians know this best. To be a joyful cook and to relish in your finished product with pride and confidence is where the magic lies.

This beginner's guide to Italian cooking can be incorporated into any lifestyle thanks to its many quick and effortless recipes that pack a punch of flavor, not to mention the jaw-dropping visuals and aromas that will impress your family and friends.

Join me on this journey and rekindle your love for fresh quality ingredients, pragmatic cooking techniques, and an overall passion for serving healthy and wholesome food.

I will be showing you how to pour in loads of love, sprinkle some inspiration, drizzle on that creativity, and whip up a marvelous creation that not only fills your belly but your soul.

Take a peek at the historical relevance of Italian cuisine, the many applications and methodologies, and of course, the 50 recipes that will be detailed in the most simplistic way possible. From starters to mains, sides, snacks, and desserts, let us jump right into the marvels of tradition and in turn its transcendence into our busy modern world.

Whether you are a newbie or a well-seasoned cook, anyone can learn how to take the stress out of the kitchen and fill that void with simplicity and laughter.

So come along and let us revel in the beauty of a country, its people, and its incredible knowledge of health in healthy cooking.

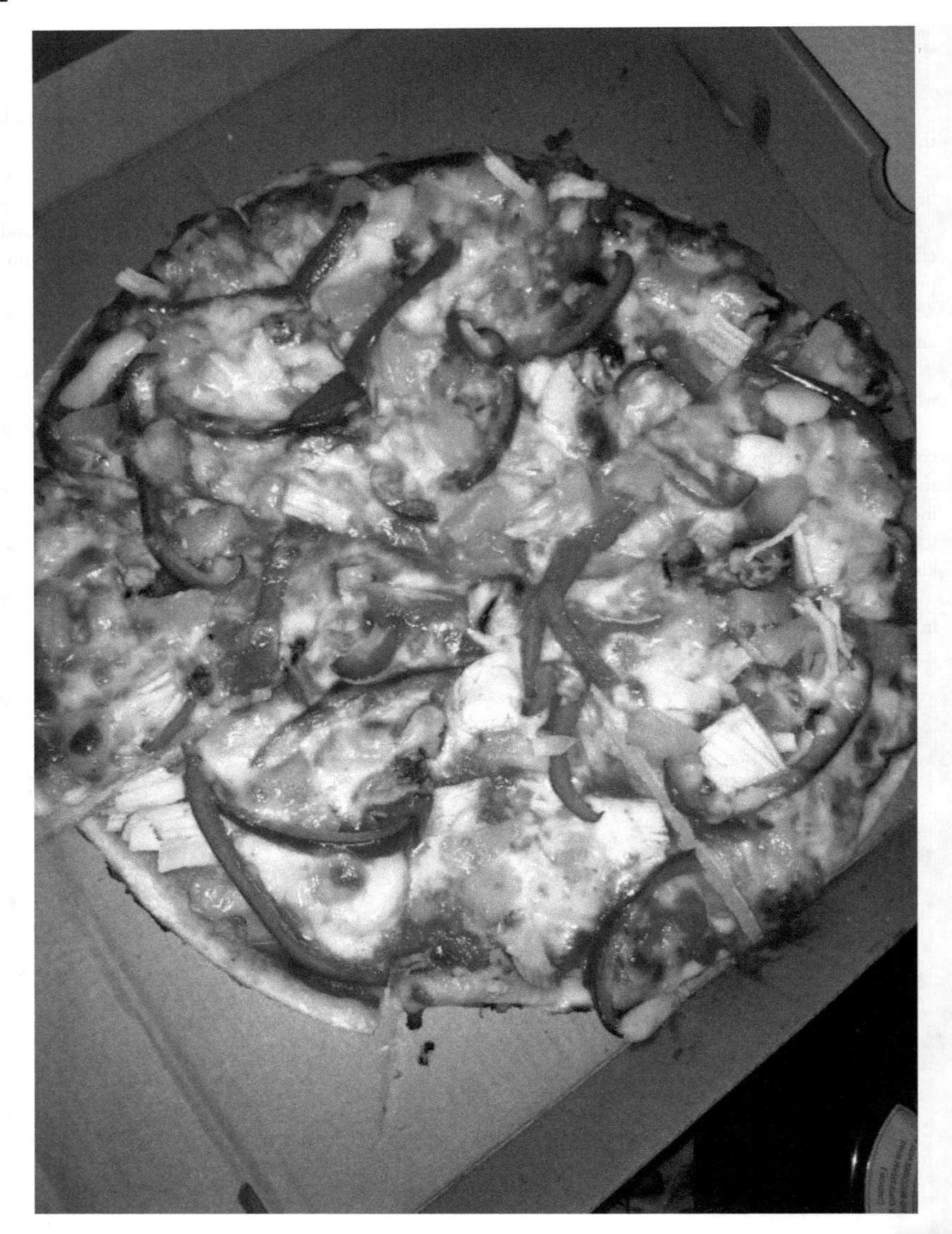

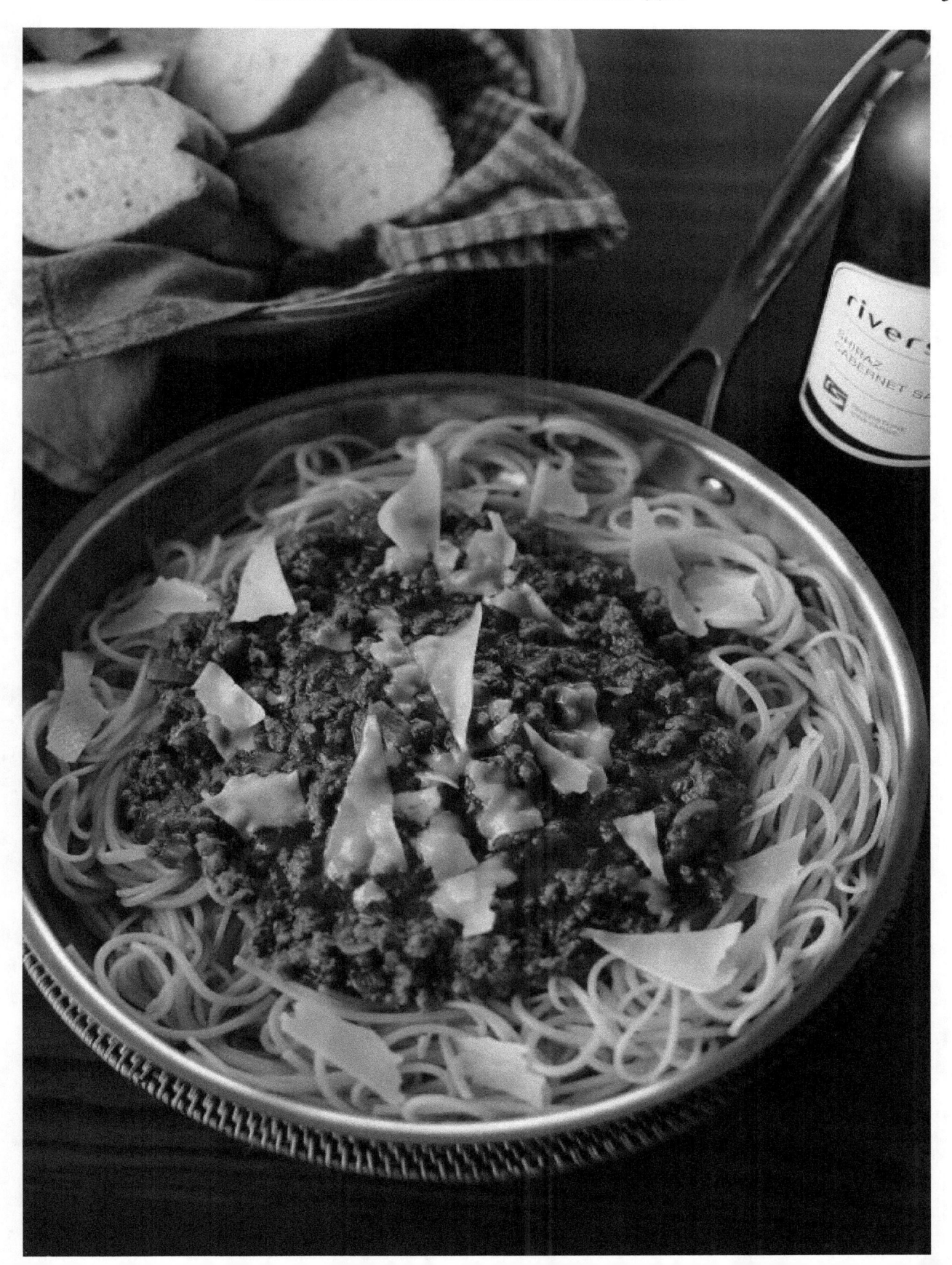

Italian Cookbook for everyday use.
Delicious and easy-to-follow Italian recipes to celebrate the cuisine the right way

ITALIAN COOKBOOK FOR EVERYDAY USE.

Maleb Briane

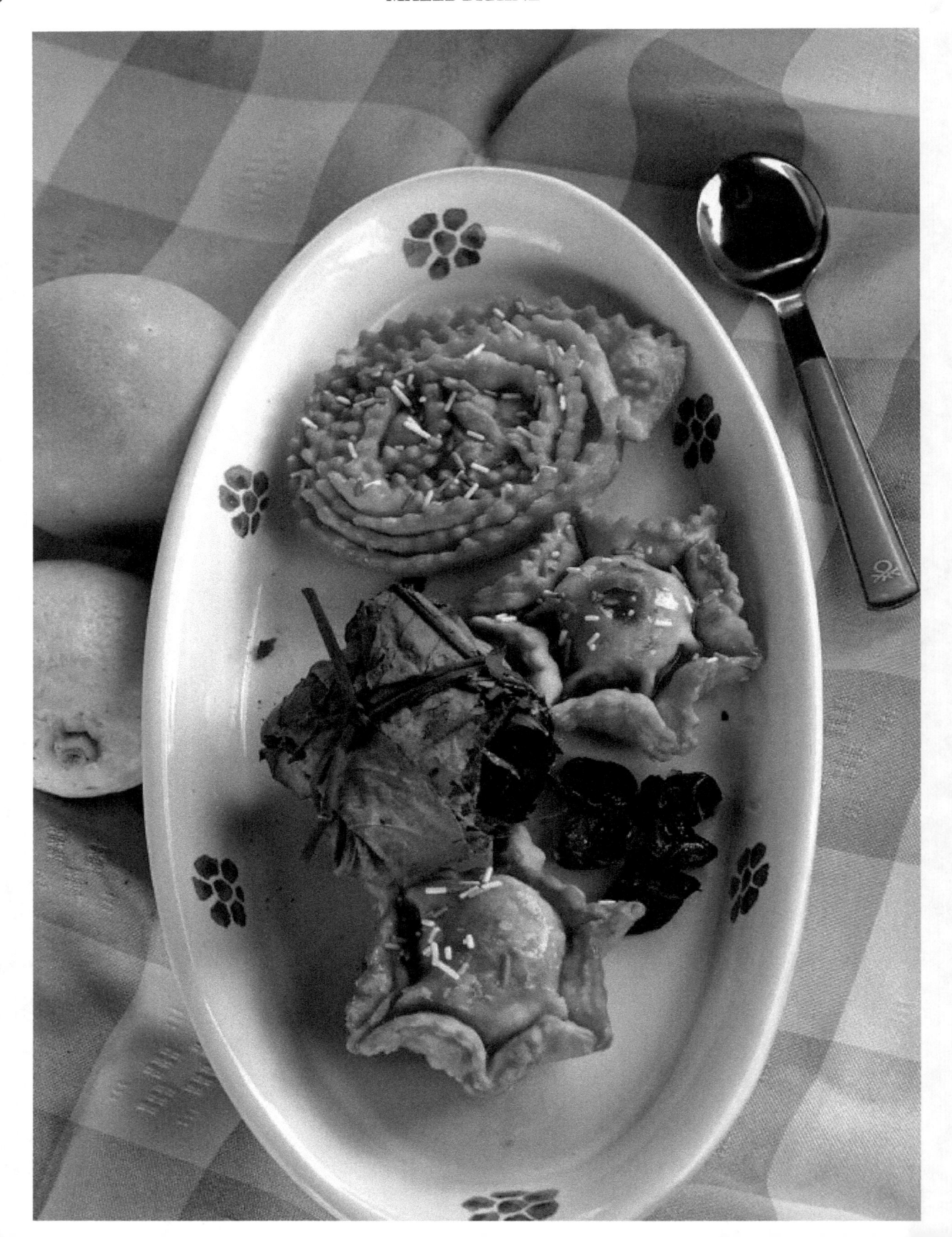

ITALIAN COOKBOOK FOR EVERYDAY USE.

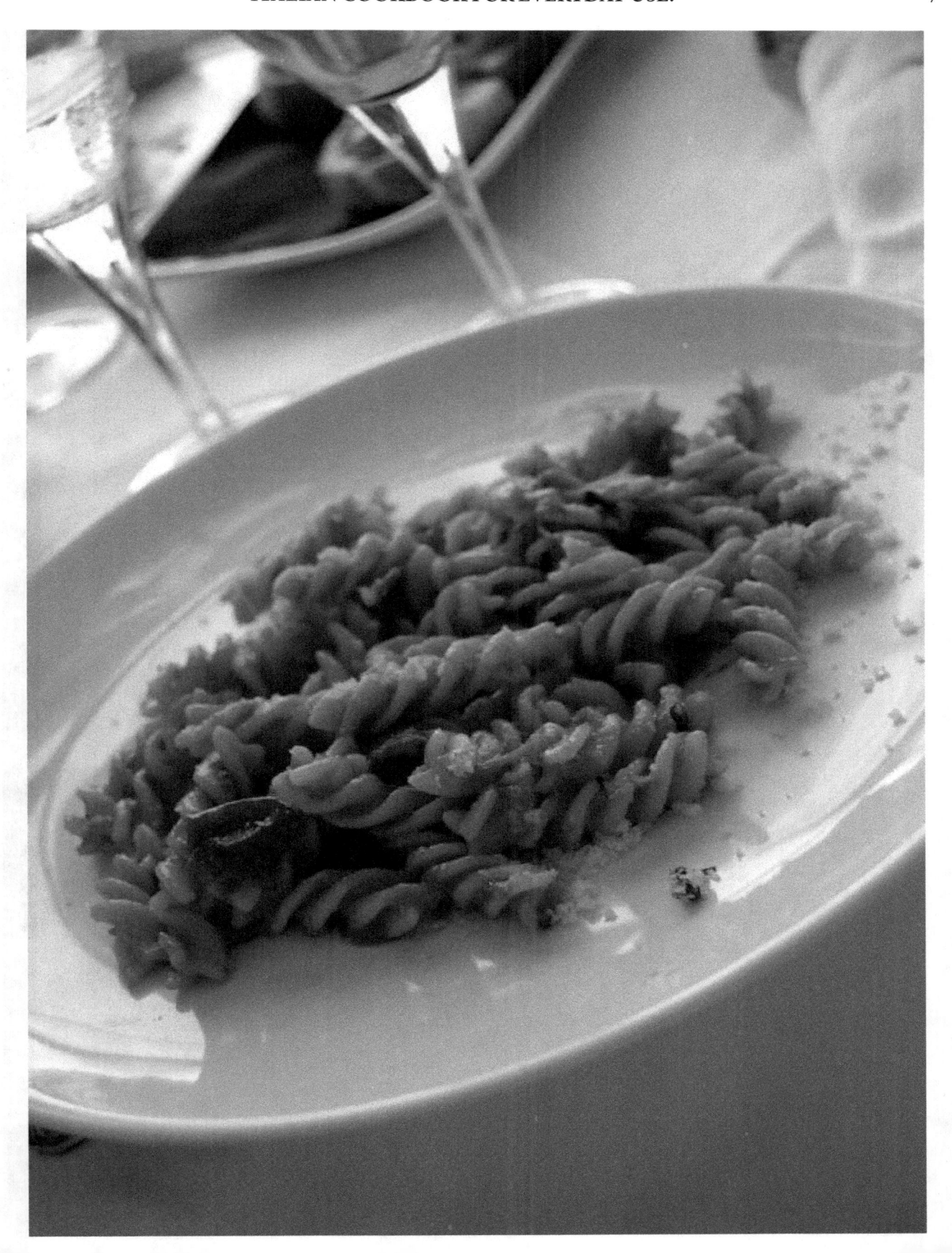

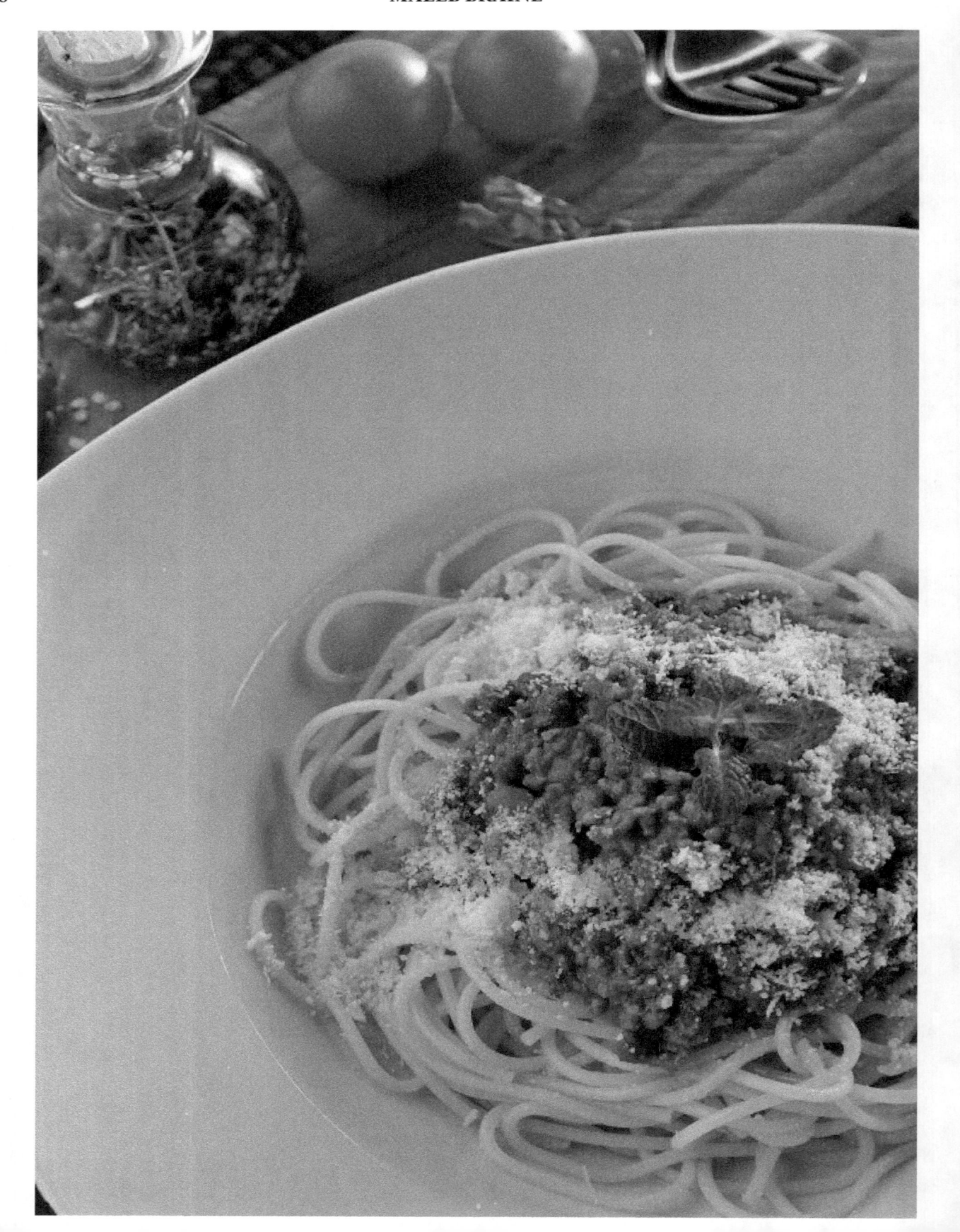

ITALIAN COOKBOOK FOR EVERYDAY USE.

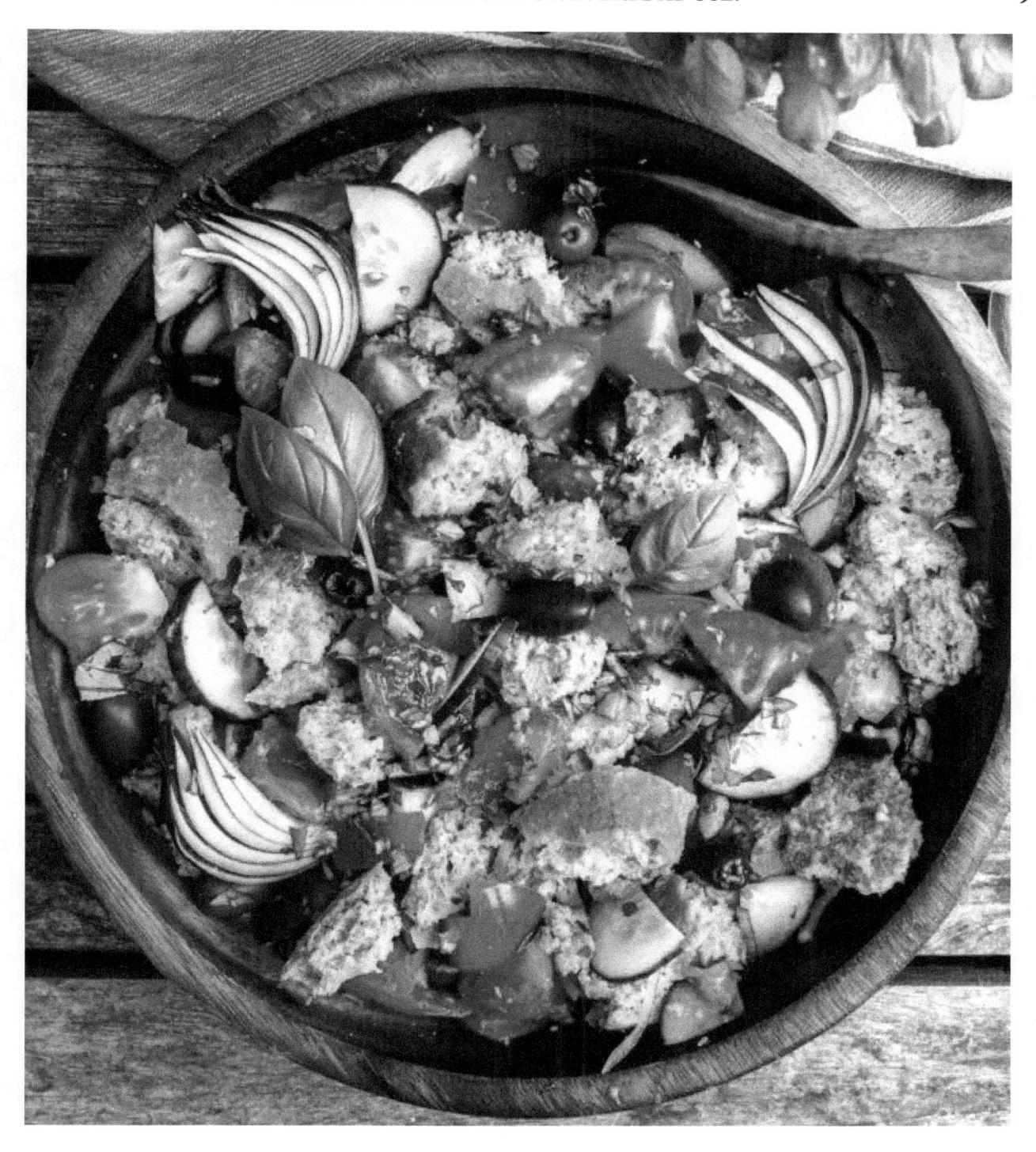

© Copyright 2022 - All rights reserved.

The content contained within this book may not be reproduced, duplicated or transmitted without direct written permission from the author or the publisher.

Under no circumstances will any blame or legal responsibility be held against the publisher, or author, for any damages, reparation, or monetary loss due to the information contained within this book, either directly or indirectly.

Legal Notice:

This book is copyright protected. It is only for personal use. You cannot amend, distribute, sell, use, quote or paraphrase any part, or the content within this book, without the consent of the author or publisher.

Disclaimer Notice:

Please note the information contained within this document is for educational and entertainment purposes only. All effort has been executed to present accurate, up to date, reliable, complete information. No warranties of any kind are declared or implied. Readers acknowledge that the author is not engaged in the rendering of legal, financial, medical or professional advice. The content within this book has been derived from various sources. Please consult a licensed professional before attempting any techniques outlined in this book.

By reading this document, the reader agrees that under no circumstances is the author responsible for any losses, direct or indirect, that are incurred as a result of the use of the information contained within this document, including, but not limited to, errors, omissions, or inaccuracies.

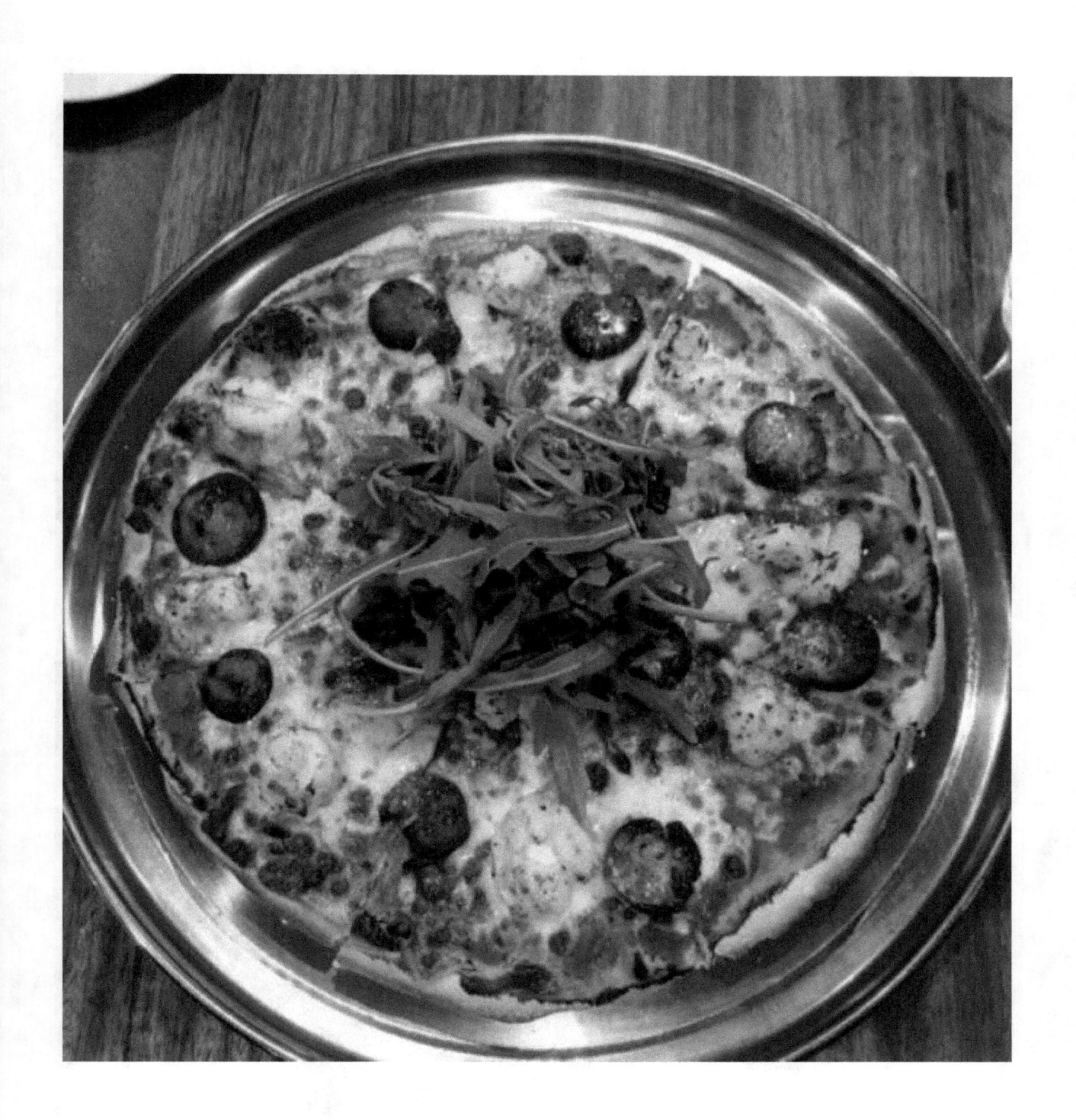

MALEB BRAINE

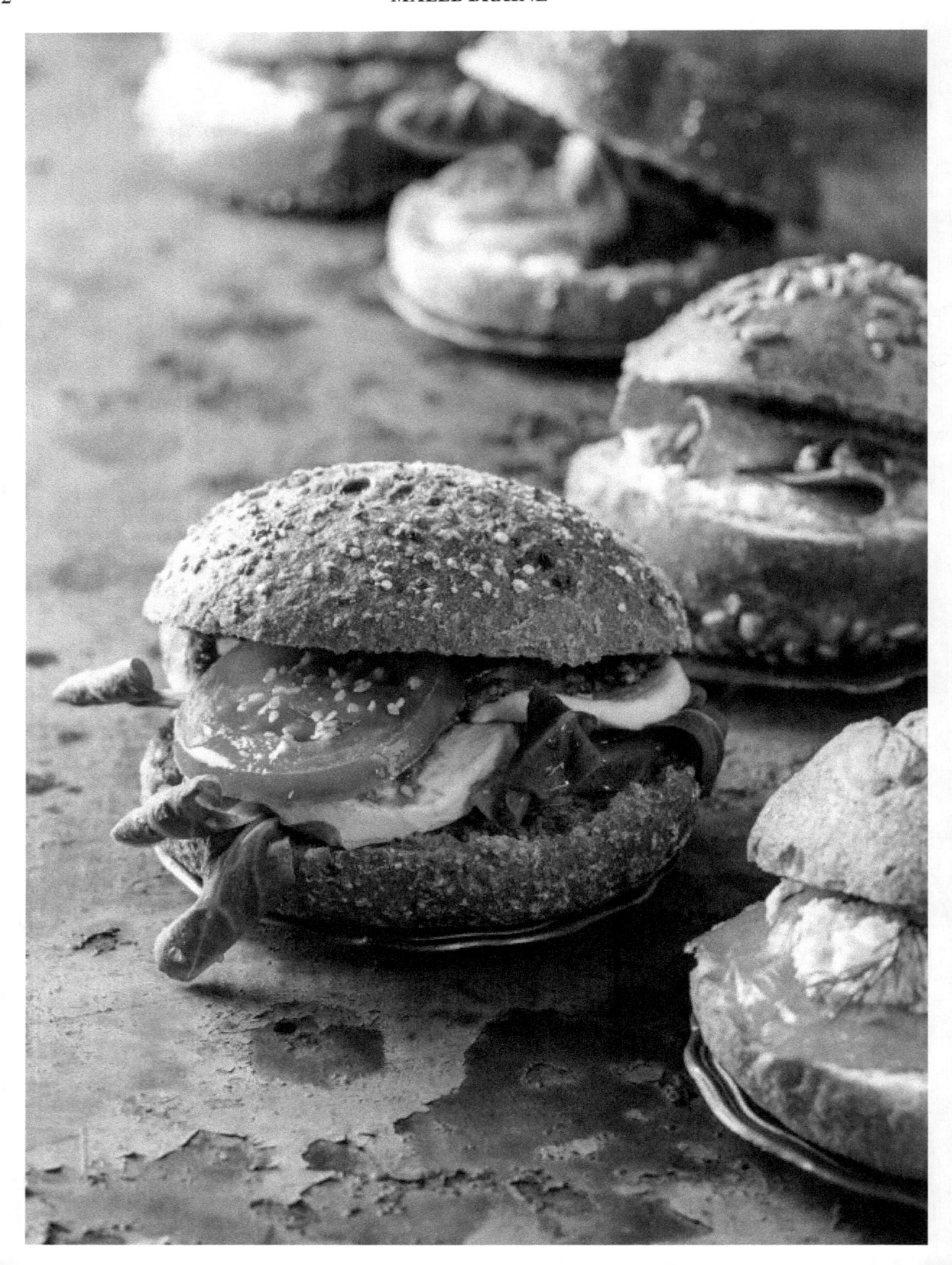

Introduction

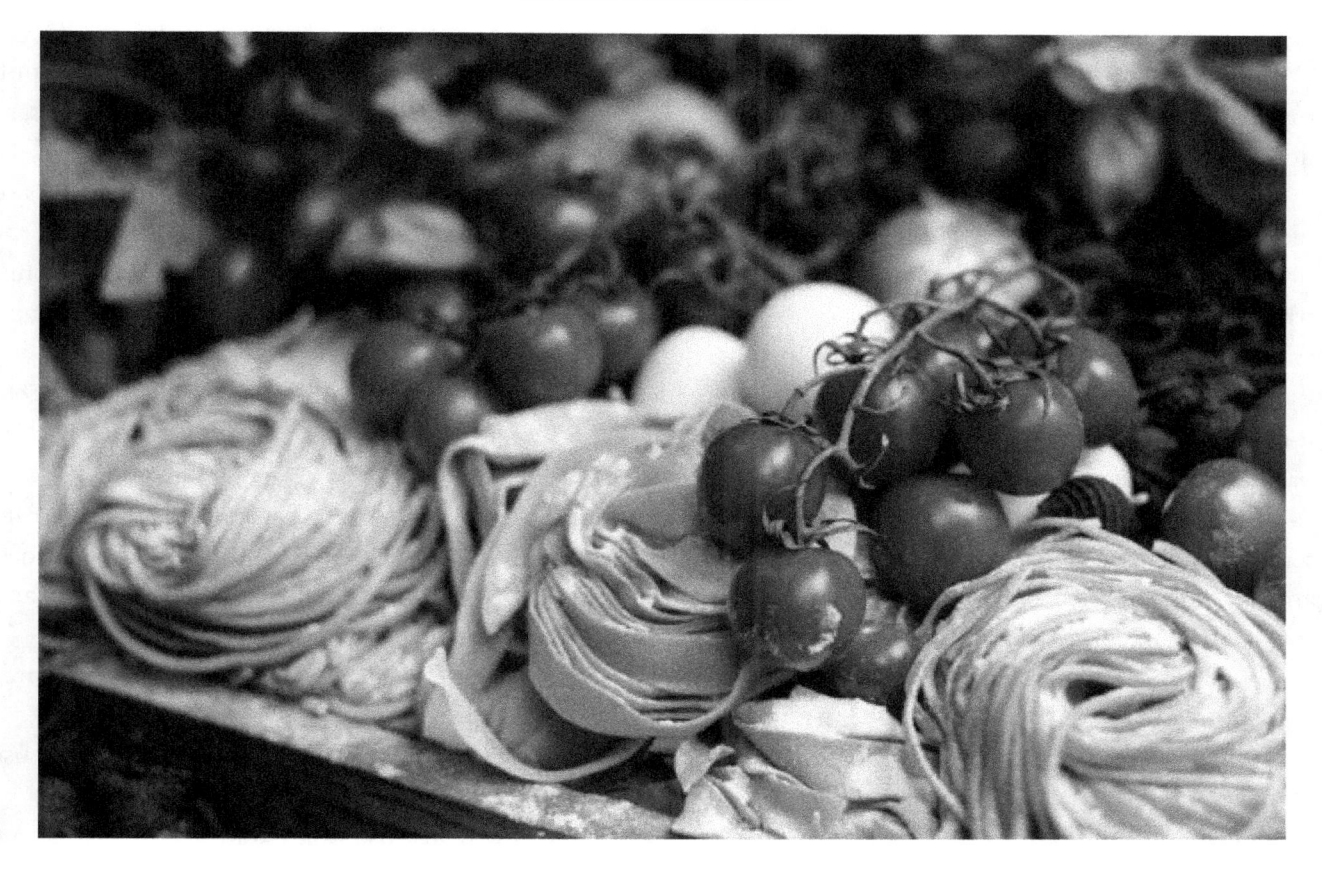

Italian food is seasonal. It is simple. It is nutritionally sound. It is flavorful. It is colorful. It's all the things that make for a good eating experience, and it's good for you. —Lidia Bastianich

The perfect Italian meal can usually be envisioned within a lush vineyard, everyone seated outside along a table under a veranda of wild grapes and buzzing insects. The sun shines through the grapevines, the red wine stains plotted across the white tablecloth, the scattered breadcrumbs residing where they were left when the bread was happily devoured by the handfuls, and of course, the empty plates scraped almost completely clean.

You do not need to see the people eating and joyfully conversing to know that something great happened here: a 6-hour lunch that turned into dinner and then a late-night festivity, a carefree and pleasure-driven atmosphere that says, "Come! Be merry and be alive. Enjoy La Dolce Vita."

The sometimes foreign but familiar concept of Italian cooking comes from the basis of living to live, not living to die, living to surround yourself with strength and vigor, where no one actually gets old, they just look a little older.

The vitality and passion in Italian cuisine are so special and unique, it almost makes you question your way of life. Should you be slowing down and remembering what is actually important rather than fussing over the trivial?

Questions like that are what connect you with something greater. And maybe, just maybe, cooking a meal from scratch, learning a new facet of cuisine, and finding the benefits of it can be life bettering or even life-altering.

Honestly, I don't think I have ever turned down an offer to eat a plate of something Italian. There is a pull towards the cuisine that many can relate to. The homeliness, the warmth, the simplicity, and the great taste cannot compare. Both the cooking and eating are meant to be fun!

That is why the "Italian way" is something of a phenomenon worldwide that transcends the differences of race, culture, age, and class. It is considered a cheaper choice of many cuisines, although far from cheap!

We see a substantial win for Italian cuisine in terms of global favorites. A gastronomical study on 24 countries surveyed in 2019 showed that a majority of that love is for Italian dishes. Is it the hearty flavor, the common and inexpensive ingredients, or the simplicity in its design?

I believe it to be a combination of all three actually. The convenience is far overshadowed by the fact that it is just so damn good! There is a saying that goes, "Italian food is like sex. When it's good, it's great. When it's bad, it's still pretty good."

Traditional Italian methods can be taxing as they usually require you to build your foundations from scratch, but in today's day and age, we can easily pop off to the store to buy the dry pasta, the canned tomatoes, and the pre-packaged fresh herbs at a reasonable price! You can make something good from the basics, and something gorgeous when you start paying attention to the simple details.

But more than being simple, it is super inclusive. You see where the flavors fit and you mold yourself accordingly, and vice versa. Expand your taste to new avenues and novel combinations.

You can learn to prepare your foundations of dough, tomato bases, and other sauces beforehand, and use them as you work through the week.

Today we find that time is short, terribly short in fact. That is why in this book I want to show you how cooking can take you away from screens, away from the noise of your daily life, and bring you back to the principles. There is so much critical thinking that you allow yourself to do when you cook. In itself, it can be self-therapy if you look at it the right way.

My intrigue really showed itself when I chose to jump the hurdle and focus my attention on what it meant to cook the Italian way. As a practicing chef and an ardent food blogger, I needed to challenge the gastronomy of Italian food so that I could show others how accommodating it actually is. As I peeled away the layers of big words, complex traditional methods, and the intricacy of sourcing the correct ingredients, I was left with a laughing Nonna (grandmother) telling me to just cook with my heart.

It is not only about the cooking, instead, it is also about what character you cook in. The more loving, respecting, and sharing you do in the kitchen, the closer you are to cooking and living the Italian way.

I am continuously surrounded by creativity, and in turn, it pushes me to be more creative and look for new ways to tell a story through food. Each ingredient has a new note or sequence in my play. When I refined the story of Italian cuisine, I was blown away by its power. It is a push and pull of tradition and practicality.

Cooking Italian cuisine is not only fun but it is a great learning curb for any beginner cook. The basics and principle methods of preparation, flavor correlation, and techniques within Italian culture will bring you tears of relief. Not to mention how popular you will be with family, friends, and colleagues!

So what exactly will you be learning in this nifty cookbook? Let's take a quick look:

Part I

- Chapter 1: The history that brought Italian cuisine to popularity

- Chapter 2: Breaking down what the taste of Italy really is

- Chapter 3: A thorough look at all the main components of Italian cuisine

- Chapter 4: The equipment needed to create a magical plate of Italian food

Part II

- Chapter 5: A deeper look at the foundations of Italian cuisine with recipes

Part III

- Chapter 6: Starters
- Chapter 7: Ricotta
- Chapter 8: Soups
- Chapter 9: Pasta
- Chapter 10: Risotto
- Chapter 11: Polenta
- Chapter 12: Pizzas
- Chapter 13: Meats
- Chapter 14: Salads
- Chapter 15: Desserts

Within each recipe from Chapter 6 to Chapter 15 I will be introducing you to various recipes in terms of cooking time estimation, serving portions, and the ingredients that will be needed. Then, we will discuss the directions to make the meal, finally followed by some nifty tips.

Please note that many ingredients that come with Italian cooking are traditional, wholesome, and natural. This means that wheat, eggs, and animal products are often used. If you are allergic to certain components or on a specific diet please be sure to look out for alternative tips in some of the recipes.

You will be amazed at what your own two hands can cook up. And you can keep that smile on your face when the compliments come flying in.

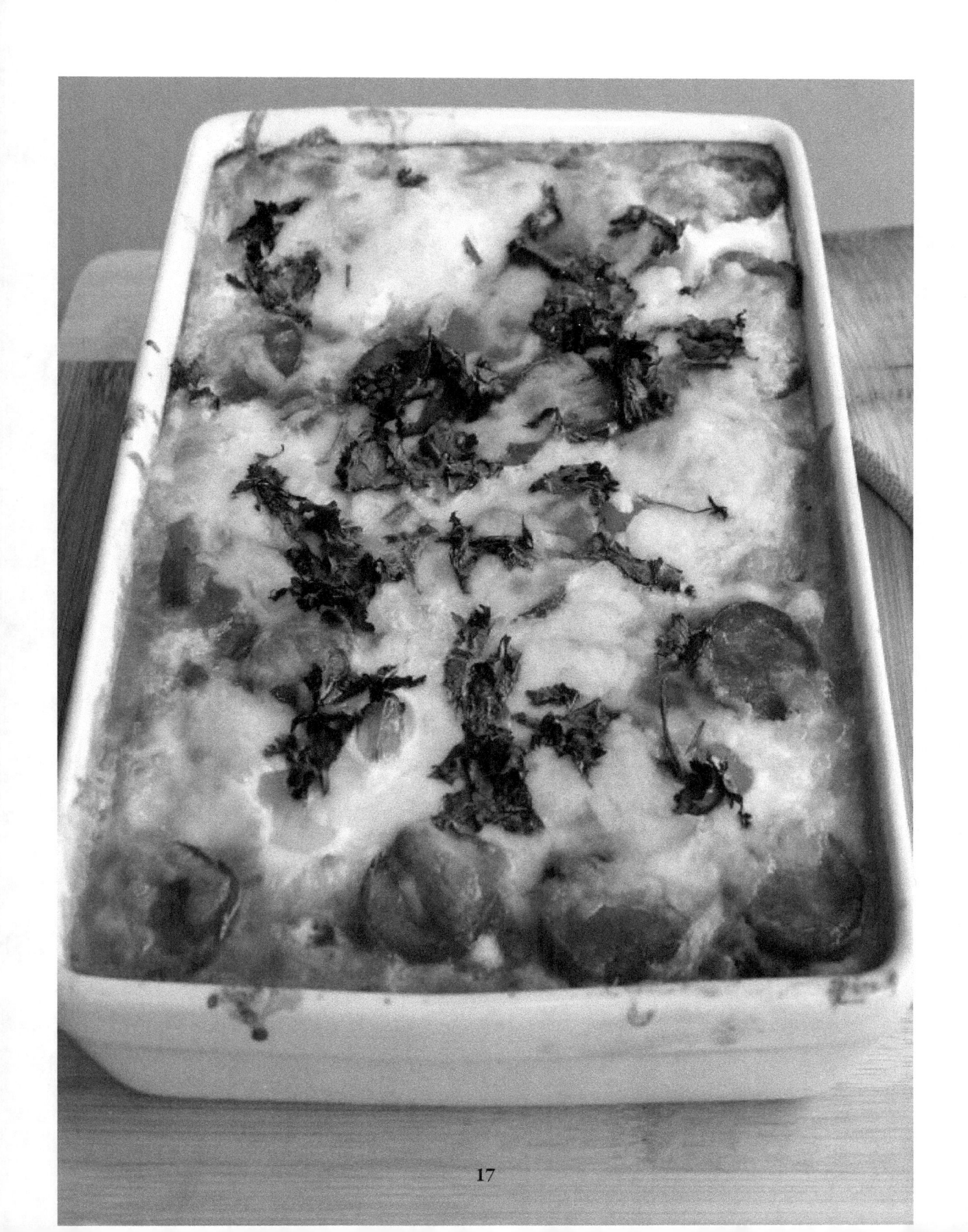

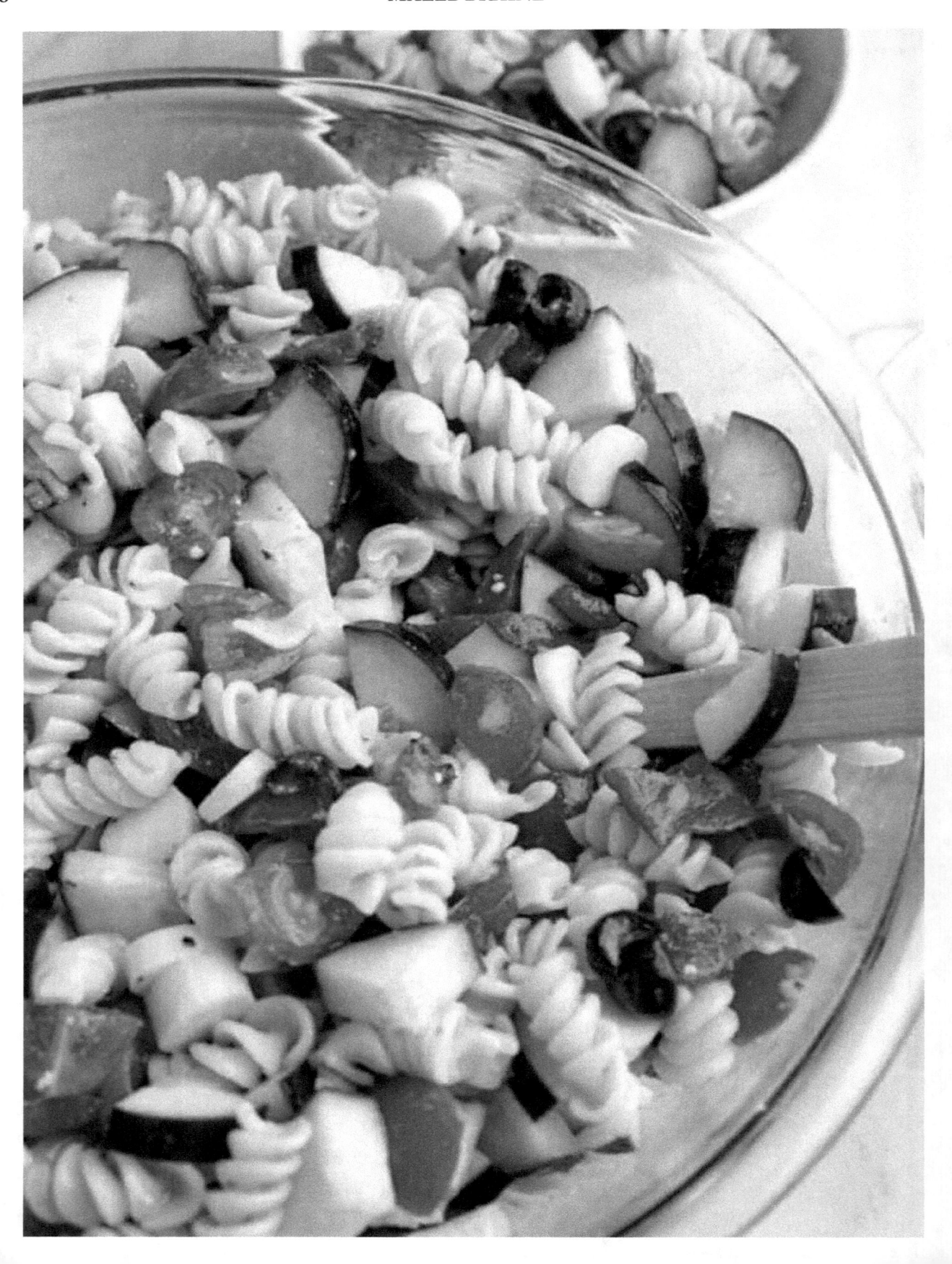

Part I - From Italy, With Love

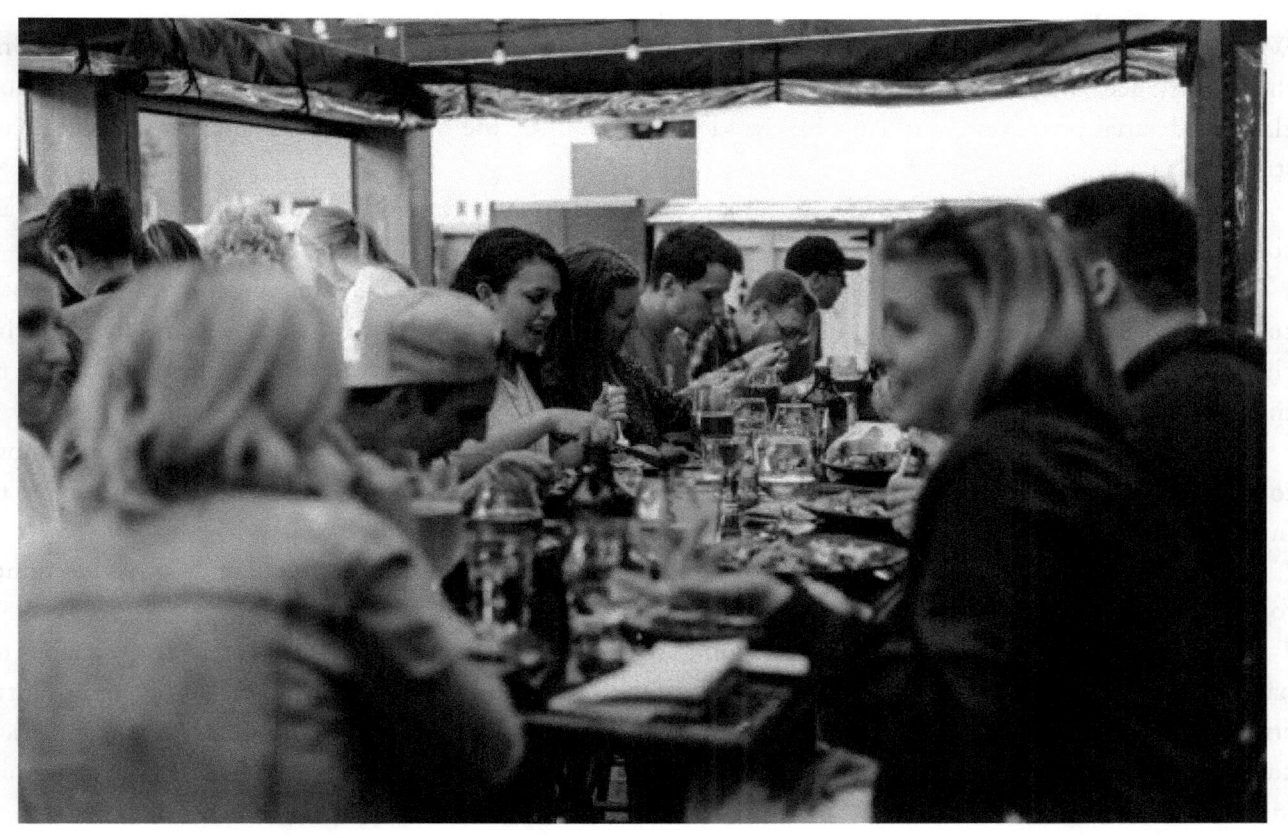

You've seen the movies and you most likely understand the romantic and sensual context of Italian culture, where cuisine is also typically portrayed. But do you know what makes Italian food so special?

In Part I, we will delve into the chapters that explain the country's style, palate, tradition, and modern takes on dishes. From its influence throughout history to its popularity in modern times, we will discover why it is such a loved cuisine all around the world.

Chapter 1: The History of Italian Cuisine

We can say that it all started in the great Roman Empire, and has evolved throughout the Middle Ages, into the Renaissance, and well into WWII: a remarkable journey into the centuries of Empirical invasion, Catholic claim, Industrial revolution, and later Fascist ideals, all molding the people, culture, and general social constructs of a nation.

The beauty shines through when you think of how this country turned its struggle into success both as a country and as a culinary masterpiece.

If you look at the geographical location alone, you can understand why Italy was able to influence an entire culinary culture. The Mediterranean climate proved bountiful through the produce of wheat, olive oil, wine, cheese, sunflowers, and a good number of fruits and vegetables that other regions of Continental Europe at the time couldn't support due to their weather and access.

The separation from the rest of Europe by the high and then sometimes impassable mountain ranges known today as the Alps was a large contender of the climate. Other pockets of islands and coastal regions pulled the influence of food widely towards the ocean.

Then we talk about their influence from and on others. Over the centuries as a Roman Empire, the country found much of its inspiration from those it conquered and those it traded with.

As the years pervaded and history did its rounds, so did the diversity of the country and its regions. The culinary vision between the north and the south of Italy started to show differences. The north leveraged the Northern European regions above it, while the south took inspiration from the Middle East and Northern African cultures residing below. Spices, meat, and cereal grain all flowed into the empire creating a hotspot for culinary infusion.

The recipes passed down from one generation to another were kept alive with pride as a way to hold onto the roots that built the nation and its template. This certainly depended on the class you were born into at the time, showing us that the noble and elite were accessing a larger variety of foods and techniques that would build the greater influence, while the peasantry sourced directly from their land, cultivating a reliance on the olive, vine, and cereal, also known as the Mediterranean Triad, or the foundation of Mediterranean cuisine.

End of the Roman Empire and Into the Middle Ages

The Romans loved many things, but what stood out was their love for banquets, festivities, and entertainment. Their consumption of fruits, cheeses, bread, and copious amounts of wine gave us the consistent image we often see today in the media.

Then, the 4th century dawned and the arrival of the Barbarians signified the end of the Roman Empire. They poured their ruggedness and simplicity into the Italian culture and in turn the cuisine. From the Roman's usual taste of grain and vine, we begin to see the inclusion of beer and butter from the Northern invaders, and the reciprocated influence of Roman olive oil and wine.

Once the Roman Empire was completely disbanded, the Catholic influence throughout the Middle Ages began to show. A subversive change in the habits and behaviors during the period saw the culture begin to distinguish more on what could and couldn't be eaten.

A culinary culture had to change from the free and fragrant ideal of the Roman Empire to the strict and pious rules that governed the culinary world after the implementation of the Catholic church. Sin, lust, and pride were all condemned, and most noticeable through culinary practices. Fasting and abstinence saw a rise as well as the exclusion of meat from the diet, as it was seen as an energetic and violent food that brought about lust and passion in an individual. Therefore, bread, legumes, grains, cheese, and seasonal fruits were more acceptable.

The Charmalagne influence in the 8th century created an equal ground between honoring the Lord and celebrating life, bringing a balance to the chastity of the Church in fasting and behaving most of the week, while keeping one or two days open for good flavors and pleasure.

In the 9th century the Arabs brought in their understanding and usefulness of dried grain, and in turn, pasta itself arrived on the shores of Italy. Its influence climbed up the boot from Sicily and eventually became incredibly popular as far as Spain and France.

Late Middle Ages and Through the Renaissance

As the 11th century dawned, the Renaissance took hold and a bourgeoisie was forming in the arts and sciences. There came a fondness for luxury and excess as a return to city life was established where people traded, built great cities, and mingled in thought and in finance. A return to the past practices of culinary freedom bloomed, and so, pleasurable food returned as a symbol of status.

The late middle ages in the north of Italy started to see a love for sugar, dried fruits, nuts, and foreign spices like cinnamon. Roasting was once more on the menu, and thanks to the Crusades opening up Europe, there was an introduction to a wider variety of fruits and vegetables.

The 13th century saw a rise in the concept of refined cooking for the nobles in their castles and villas. A far more conservative way of cooking took hold that elevated chefs and in turn food to newer heights of grandiosity. Even though still simple, the methods that were introduced changed Italian cooking forever.

From the Arabs, in the south of Italy, we see lemons, sugar cane, and almonds flow inland. And here comes the big one: gelato, or traditional Italian ice cream, is said to originate from this combination of Sicilian and Arabic taste.

As the 14th and 15th century showed up, so did the palate for gastronomical experimentation. Gourmet bread filled with nuts, honey, and dried fruits. More intricate methods evolved in the kitchen with professional chefs experimenting with techniques like frying and pickling. At this time, the invention of filled pasta took place and the inclusion of more tomato products in the 17th century brought forth the invention of pizza and the use of boiling dried pasta and adding tomatoes on top.

Through the Industrial Revolution

There was a fierce rivalry between the French delicacy of cooking and that of Italian food, which some might say still persists today (not only in cuisine). The shape and form of Italian cuisine came into their own.

The creation of tiramsú came about around this time as well, along with other very delicate and intricate desserts. As people began to travel with more ease, so did ingredients. Italian food could now be exported and began influencing the rest of the world.

In the mid 17th century, we see the first modern cookbook being published by a Neapolitan chef. Detailed descriptions of novel methods of cooking, intricate recipes, and ingredient resourcing were a fantastic accomplishment for the time.

But as the 19th century dawned, so did the value of Italy as a whole; it was a country coming out of struggle and repression in all shapes and forms, finally free to move forward.

Into Modernity

From the 20th century, we see a congregation of the regional differences of Italian cuisine. Internally, Italians distinguished their regional foods with pride, but now they were starting to see that maybe they should portray a cuisine that was one entity to the rest of the world instead of its regional disputing cuisines.

Recipe books started to pop up with the inclusion of southern and northern dishes, along with new inventions and applications. Every new year brought new discoveries in gastronomy.

Through both WWI and WWII, food became scarce and heavily rationed. The staple of pasta and rice was the easiest and cheapest option and people became frugal, although as you would expect, the Italian forces always seemed to have better food than the rest of Europe's troops. Unsurprisingly, around this time, canned goods became major players, infiltrating the market for good.

After the wars, an immersion of food and art took hold in Italy, where people were showing flair like never before in tradition, pride, and patriotism to their food and culture. What we know today of traditional Italian food started taking shape during this time with a return to normal life, an increase in economy, and the help of importing and exporting produce.

An understanding of slow-cooked foods occurred. In equal measure, women were entering the workforce and that meant less time spent in the kitchen. Italians started looking for faster ways to get the same food, but without compromising quality.

As the centuries passed, rules were broken, new methods were created, novel combinations were brought forth, and a newfound passion for food was born that still follows Italians to this day.

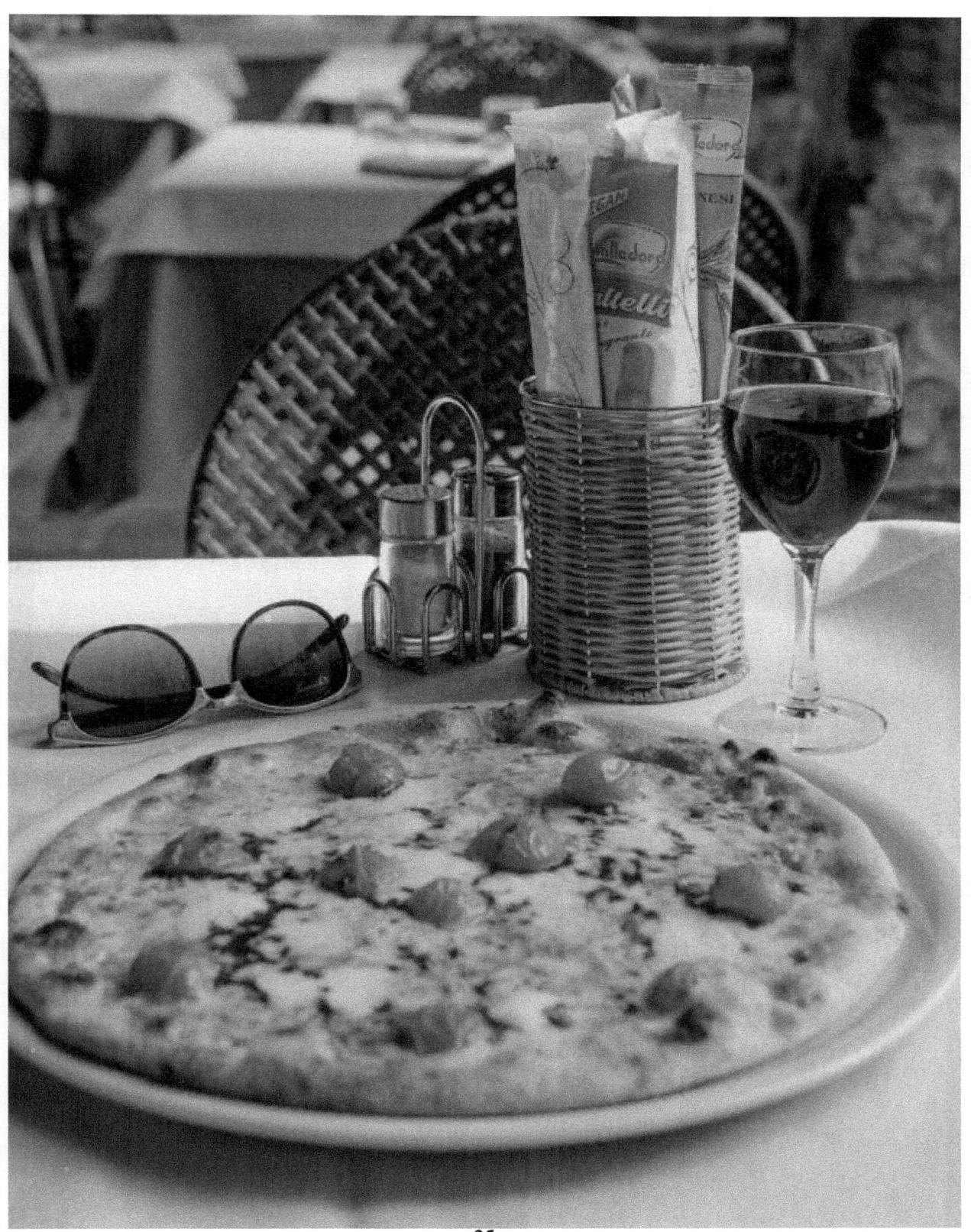

Chapter 2: A Taste of Culture

The taste of Italy is not merely the taste of a culture, but the taste of times when work was done by hand and when time flowed slowly as the sun grazed the skies.

The base ingredients we take for granted today were laboriously processed by hand, an effort and love imbued into the essence of that product.

Recipes were honed and a life was built within a kitchen, the busiest place in the house. Women cooked together, gossiping, laughing, and crying. Pride and power come from being in the kitchen and feeding your family and history was taught within it too.

Powerful and creative ideals bloomed and recipes grew. First the mothers, sisters, and daughters, then as time passed, sons, brothers, and fathers also found their joy in cooking.

Cooking and eating is where everyone is on the same level, a place to share food and thoughts, to be merry and invested in one another. Food was appreciated because it was understood what it took to get it on the table. The longer the people spent conversing, the longer they honored that meal.

I believe the value of Italian culture has traveled the world, this culture of pleasure over pain, quality over quantity, and simplicity above all. That is not to say that Italian cuisine cannot be complex and refined, like French cuisine, but that does not take away from the greater good it brings people when they cook and eat Italian food.

The emotional balance of duty and desire is a great effector on other cultures who enjoy Italian cuisine. Lovingly coming together to eat was sharing something greater than the food itself.

Let us look at the core principles of Italian cuisine:

Tradition

There is no school like the old school and Italians seem to understand this better than most. There is a fast-paced atmosphere within first-world countries today, making it even more noticeable how Italy prefers to take it slow. Incredibly proud of tradition, their passion shines the brightest through their cuisine.

Simplicity

You live and die by the simple rule of life: don't overthink it! Take steps to ease the mind and relax into a practical application of foodstuffs. Working with a broad spectrum of quality ingredients means that you do not have to go out of your way to make a meal.

The trick here is to remember where your priority lies. Like they say, "Keep it simple, stupid." Basic ingredients that are bought with care and are used with purpose, tools that are maintained and looked after so that they may assist in making these great meals, and just knowing when to start something and when to wait is the key. Sounds simple right?

Freshness

The fresher the ingredients, the more energy, flavor, and vigor the meal holds. Frozen food products were not a common sight in a typical Italian household until the late 20th century. Freshness was the way Italian cuisine unlocked such richness.

For example, the use of tomatoes and cheese is a major game player within the cuisine. Both are incredibly simple ingredients, but when bought well, and used well, something so simple can become something beautiful. It just takes some training to get the right eye for when, where, and how much to use, but the truth is you can never go wrong with something fresh.

You have limited time to use food and that means that you have to plan well ahead of your meal. Fresh and crispy ingredients will change your life if you let them.

Authentic

One cannot pinpoint a single cuisine that is 100% authentic. Influence is everything to humankind and that is how we have come to be today. But when we look at how cuisine might have changed in different cultures as they were growing and dying, then we can see that Italian cuisine has changed very little over the centuries.

This is not to say that it has not evolved into modern cuisine, but that it has managed to keep its authentic style over all these years without being overly influenced by others, retaining a method and value to patience, quality, and love in everything they do.

Italian cuisine is a unique and intriguing gastronomical space that has been honored and honed to perfection.

Healthy

Italian food has a wonderful conundrum to its disposition as being both a healthy choice as well as comfort food. There seems to be a misconception that comfort equals unhealthy. But that does not hold water in Italian cuisine. This is because we are talking about healthy traditional dishes, not just heavy pasta and thick pizzas that we know in Western culture. There is more than just the rich sauces, starchy and gluten-packed pastas, and decadent ice creams.

Italy is certainly low in terms of obesity levels worldwide. So why do we see these starchy meals as unhealthy? Why is it that when you go on a diet, the first thing people say is to stay away from Italian food?

The answer comes with the amount Italians eat. They allow the energy from quality ingredients to build their day, eating at specific times, and at regular portions. Dinners last long, but they do not overeat, it is in the conversation around the regular amount of food on the table that keeps Italians there.

Italians indulge in small amounts, eating within their limit and thus not gaining excessive weight. Eat whatever you like, just eat wisely!

Chapter 3: The Core Ingredients

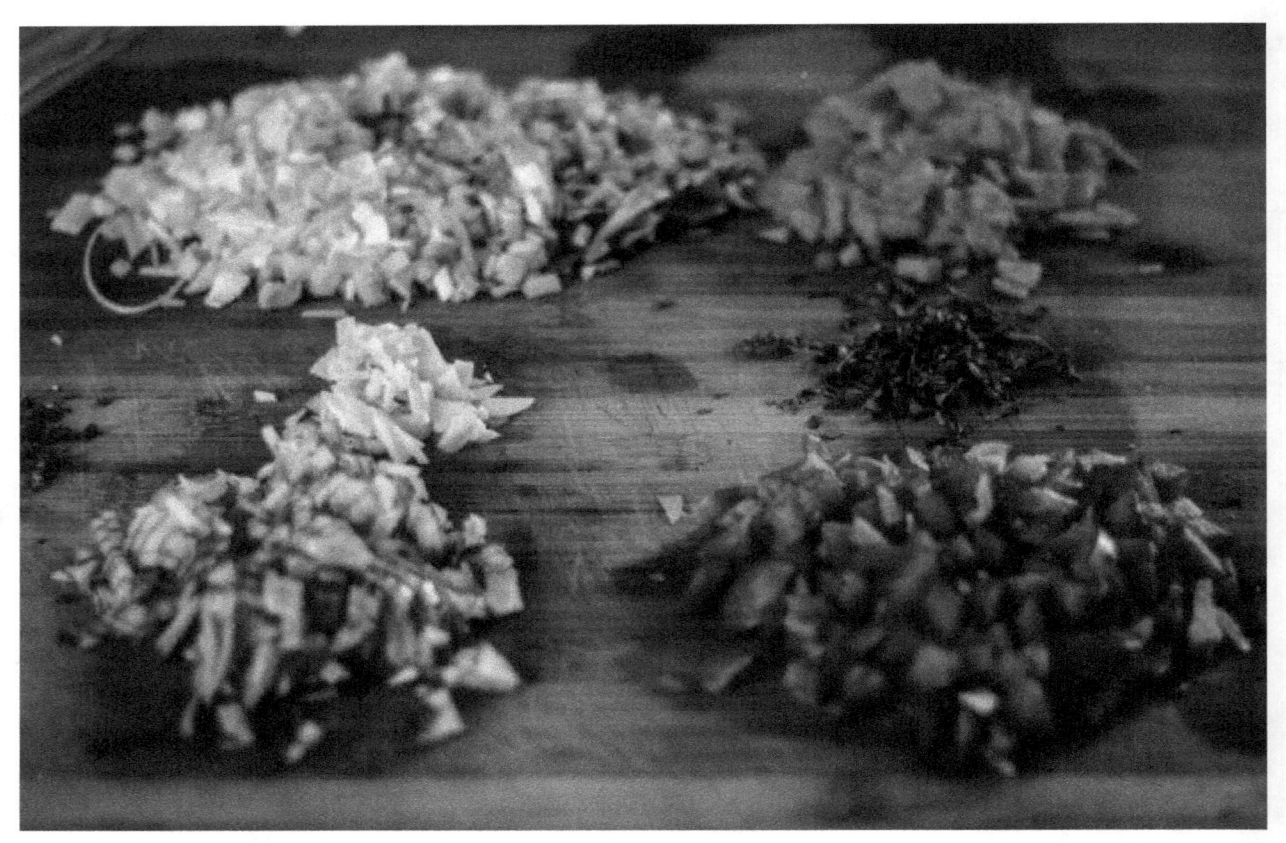

When you are dealing with authentic Italian cuisine, then you will be happy to know that the ingredients rarely change. The basics are simple, and the fresher the ingredients are, the better.

The pantry and fridge are sacred. They should be stocked well.

Let us have a good look at what the core ingredients consist of and how you can mold it to your lifestyle and tastes.

Flours and Other Grains

Pasta and bread are always present in an Italian pantry. This can be either store bought or made by hand using various kinds of pasta flours like semolina and 00 (double zero) flour. Even though all-purpose flour is used, there is more need for a specialized flavor in certain dishes.

What is the difference you might ask? AP flour is a lighter and more universal flour that bakes well with standard recipes, while semolina and 00 are denser and create a tougher and crispier texture to the bread or pasta. Semolina is very coarse and perfect for pasta, while 00 has more refined and perfect for pizza.

Breadcrumbs are used frequently to bread and hold certain dishes together when cooking. Some meals call for fresh breadcrumbs, while others need something a little stale. Yes, stale bread has its specific uses and if you travel to Italy, you will find that you can purchase fresh bread as well as a couple of free loaves of last week's bread.

Polenta is yellow cornmeal that can be eaten as a sweet or savory porridge or compressed into a compacted shape. Perfect for soaking up sauces and beautifully gluten-free.

Aromatics

Onions, garlic, carrots, parsley, and celery are aromatics. I mean, this is just so easy, right?

What gets me the most excited about eating is the first 10 minutes of cooking, when you have chopped your onions, sliced your garlic, and they are sauteing in a pan of olive oil. Now that smell is killer! It switches on something in your brain that says, "Food time!"

These vegetables are brilliant base ingredients that you will find should never be too far from your everyday meal prep.

Healthy Fats

Olive oil for days guys! Whether extra virgin or not, this is the lifeforce of Italian food. Sometimes just a drizzle, sometimes a lot more than that; you will notice that you simply cannot go without it.

Extra virgin olive oil (EVOO) is a lot more refined and delicate, with its cold-pressed olives carrying greater vitamins and antioxidants, whereas normal olive oil you often see at a cheaper price in stores is a combination of both EVOO and normal oil which retains less beneficial elements.

EVOO does not always do well at high temperatures, therefore be sure to use combination olive oil for cooking, and EVOO for dressing and flavoring meals.

Butter is often used too in Italian cooking but less often.

Seasoning

Salt and pepper are in almost all meals: kosher salt, sea salt, fine salt, coarse salt, ground black pepper, whole black pepper, and white pepper.

You will not see the use of as many spices as, let's say, Indian cuisine, because Italians find more regard for their flavors through the freshness and base products.

Fresh Herbs and Vegetables

These consist of thyme, basil, rosemary, oregano, coriander, sage, and chives. Italians will often be seen with a small herb garden in their backyards or on their porches.

These herbs add a touch of intrigue to the meal, both in their implementation of cooking under heat as well as their value as a garnish. Chopped, sliced, or added in whole, these little guys will become your best friends when you start appreciating the amount of flavor they actually imbue into each meal. Just be sure to not overdo it.

The same goes for eggplant, lemons, and tomatoes, which when added fresh to a meal can greatly increase the flavor and texture.

Vinegars

Balsamic vinegar is an invigorating component to many meals. appreciated for its unique acidity and sweetness and minimizing the need to over salt.

White vinegar uses the same principles, except we see this more in the actual process of cooking because vinegar balances out the flavors of the meats and vegetables well.

Many Italians keep a bottle of cooking wine close to the stove for those exact moments of needed balance. I mean, wine is just a fun version of normal vinegar!

Canned and Jarred Goods

This includes canned goods like whole tomatoes, crushed tomatoes, roasted tomatoes, chopped tomatoes, and many more. You might see tomato paste sachets that bring a concentrate to the dish.

Canned fish like anchovies and canned beans are common too.

Jarred products like capers, artichokes, olives, and asparagus are keenly used in the cuisine. Sure, you could very well go buy these fresh, but who always has the time? Not to mention the oil, herbs, and spices that are added into the jars and cans that make sure that the produce has even more flavor.

Cheese

You would never catch an Italian without any cheese in the house. From hard cheeses that get grated over nearly everything to soft cheeses that are incorporated into bigger meals, cheese is a winner!

Dairy products along with eggs are required in most of the recipes, so it would be valuable for someone who isn't familiar with the taste and use of the various Italian cheeses to start to get to know the flavors and test each with a curious palate.

Cured Meats

Prosciutto, salumi, or pancetta (bacon) pack a lot of flavor into a small portion. Meat brings a sense of character to the meal, but they are not the meal. Small portions of cured meats are a conscious way to eat, elevating the overall meal but not overpowering it.

Broth and Stock

Used widely in many Italian dishes, the subtle and hearty flavor of stock or broth can maximize any meal. A broth is a vegetable or meat "water," meaning that you have let vegetables or fleshy meat boil in water for some time; you can then use that broth in other dishes or eat it as is.

Stock on the other hand is made from boiling down chicken, beef, or fish bones. It is far richer and great to add when wanting to pack flavor and color into your cooking.

Wine

Seriously, who doesn't like cooking with a nice big glass of wine? Sometimes I feel that I cannot concentrate without it. Cue the curious looks.

But really, one hand holding a glass of wine, the other stirring the sauce, turning the meat, checking the pasta. It all comes down to the fact that one should be invested in having fun in the kitchen!

Red or white, you learn to cook with it and you learn to cook while drinking it. Red works best with heavy meats, while white plays well with lighter and more complex meals of fish and chicken. But hey! No need to complicate it. Whatever color you like best, just make sure to keep it stocked up.

Coffee

Coffee is life. And just like wine, it is both used to elevate a dish, mostly desserts, and it is consumed as is to wake up and get the days started.

　　Italians especially tend to enjoy smaller coffees like espresso made in a Mocha machine on the stovetop as a quick pick me up for a long and busy day.

Sparkling Water

Italians love bottled water. The main reason is that their natural tap water is not always palatable. High concentrations of chlorine and a hard taste make it difficult to drink, so drinking bottled water, specifically sparkling water, is their go-to.

Sparkling water also has many uses in dishes. Sparkling water brings aeration to batters and can be added to wine to bring more, well, sparkle!

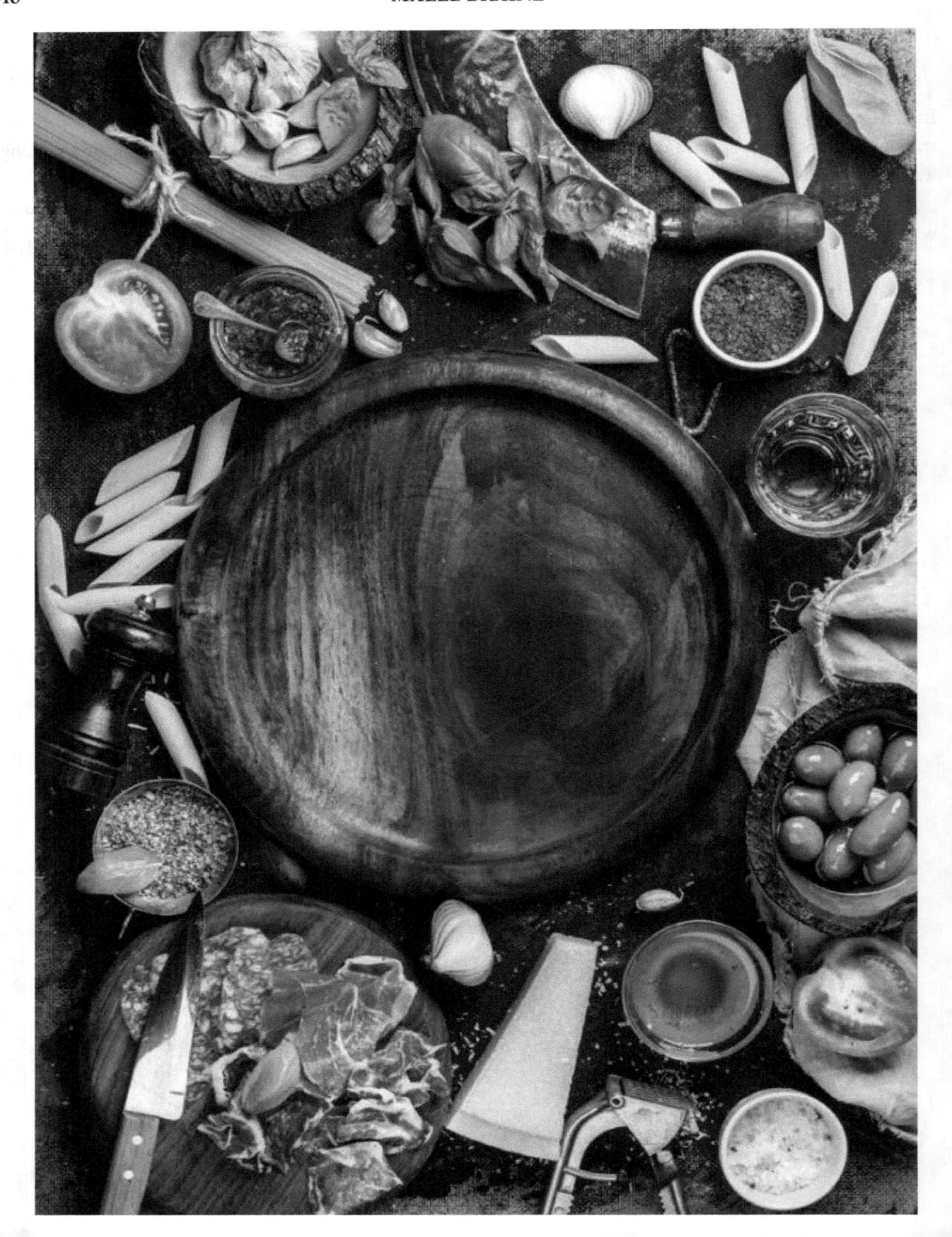

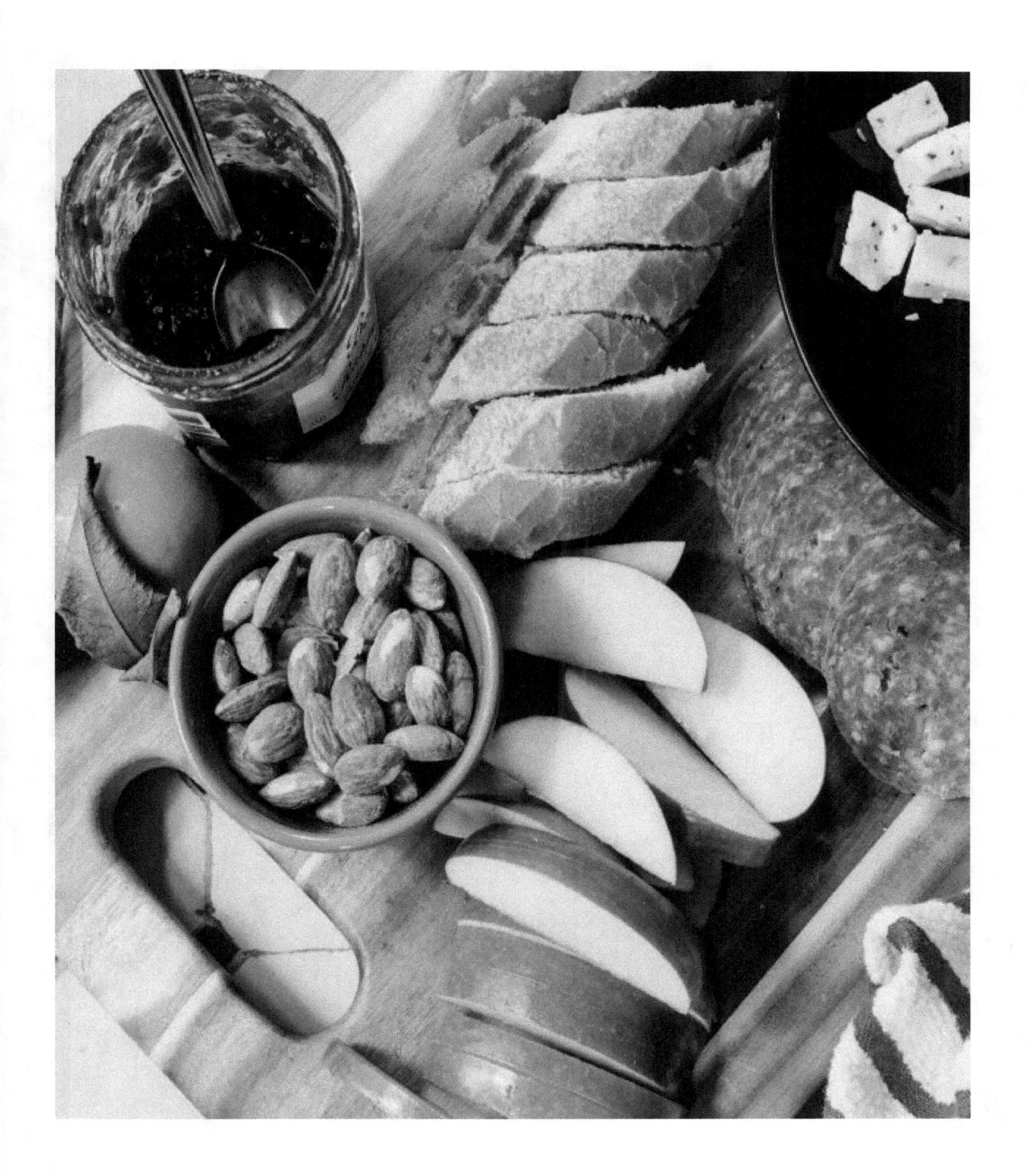

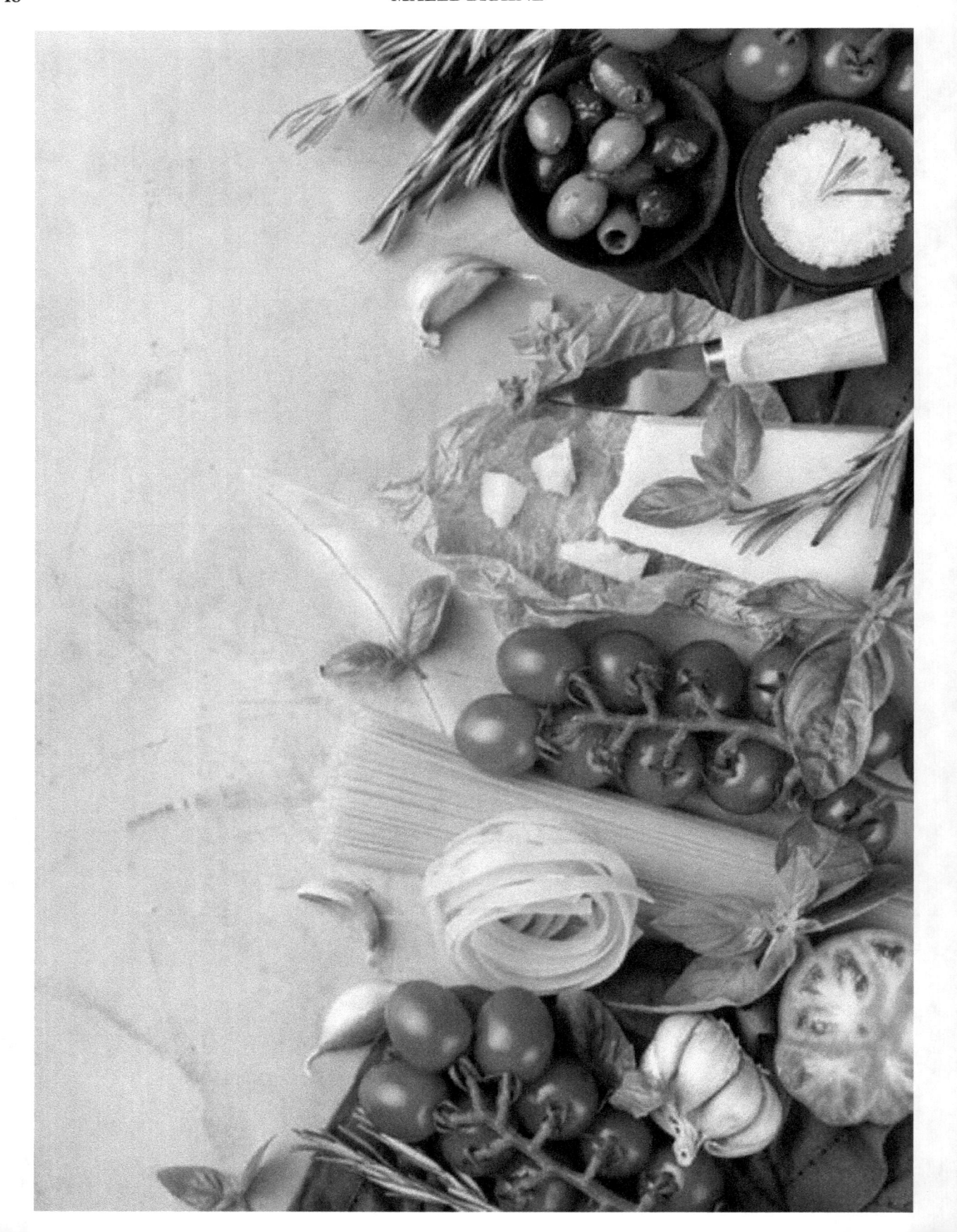

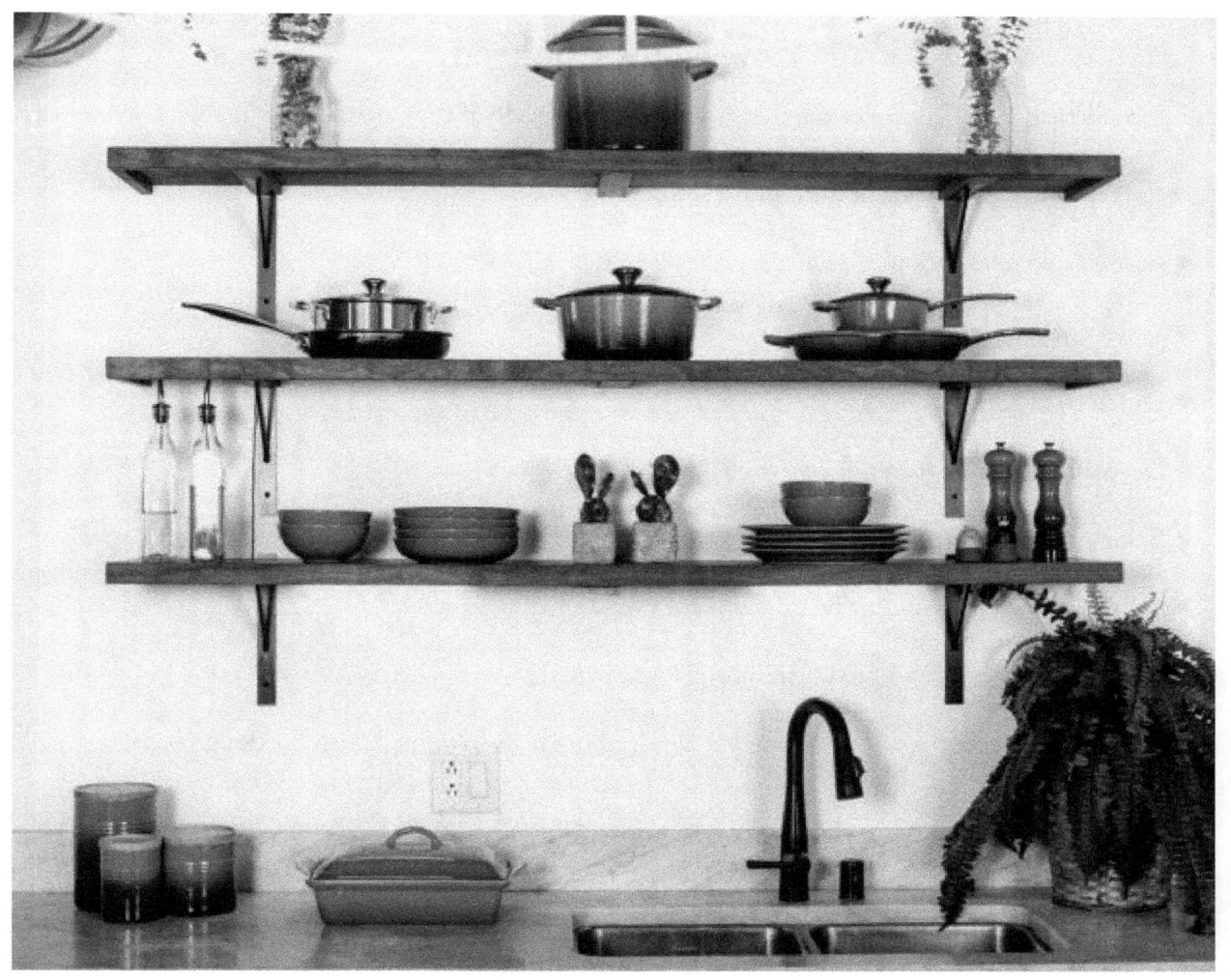

Chapter 4: Equipping Your Kitchen

If you are using the right equipment, then you are halfway there. To where you may ask? Well, to the place where you see yourself flowing around your kitchen with ease and comfort, confident in your tools and in your techniques.

Let us have a good look at what these tools may be and what they are used for specifically to increase your skills in the kitchen.

Consistent Cookware

It is important that you take care of the things you own, especially if they are of good quality. I always say, one good pan and one good knife can make a chef out of anyone.

Let us take a very quick look at the equipment needed:

- At least two non-stick pans (saucepans, frying pans, skillets)

- Variety of pots (small, medium, and large)

- Dutch oven (ceramic or cast iron)

- Deep baking dishes (ceramic or pyrex)

- Baking trays (both rimmed and flat)

- At least two large chopping boards (one for meat, one for vegetables)

- Food mill (mashing and mixing in mushy ingredients)

- Pizza stone (a ceramic or metal slab that is placed in the oven to help crisp the dough base)

Useful Utensils

- Quality vegetable and meat knives (mezzaluna knife, parmesan knife, and more)

- Slotted spoon (a must for pasta as it retrieves from water well)

- Mortar and pestle (a more traditional way to crush and mix ingredients)

- Grater and garlic press (these are extremely helpful in doing a great job in half the time)

- Colander (straining your pasta, duh)

- Tongs (easier to handle pasta and toss in with sauce of choice)

- Baking paper (for preventing the foods sticking to the baking tray when baking)

- Rolling pin (a larger rolling pin can make your life a lot easier)

- Oil and vinegar decanters (measuring carefully how much is used and making it far easier to serve)

- Pizza cutter (well, how else are you gonna get those slices out?)

- Immersion blender (these handheld blenders are perfect to blitz vegetables together in no time)

- Quality drying cloths (drying washed vegetables, and keeping fresh pastas from sticking)

Specifics

- Pasta machine (an important tool in the kitchen to create the perfect length and width of pasta)

- Pasta stand (one needs to dry the pasta properly before storage)

- Ravioli cutter (these are molds that cut out the pasta into shapes)

- Moka stovetop coffee machine (as mentioned above, Italian coffee needs one of these)

- Gnocchi board (used to roll out your gnocchi balls into the typical gnocchi shape)

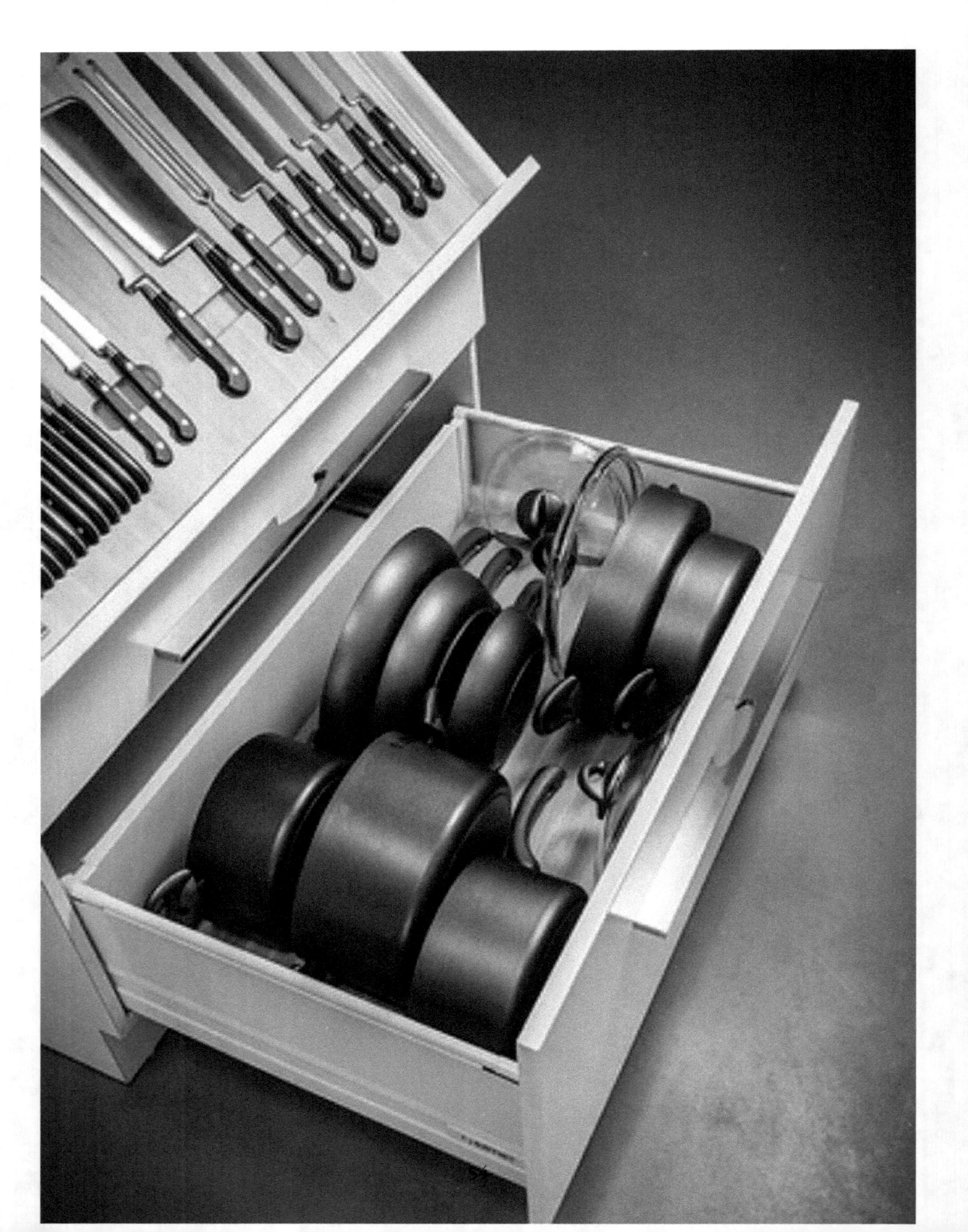

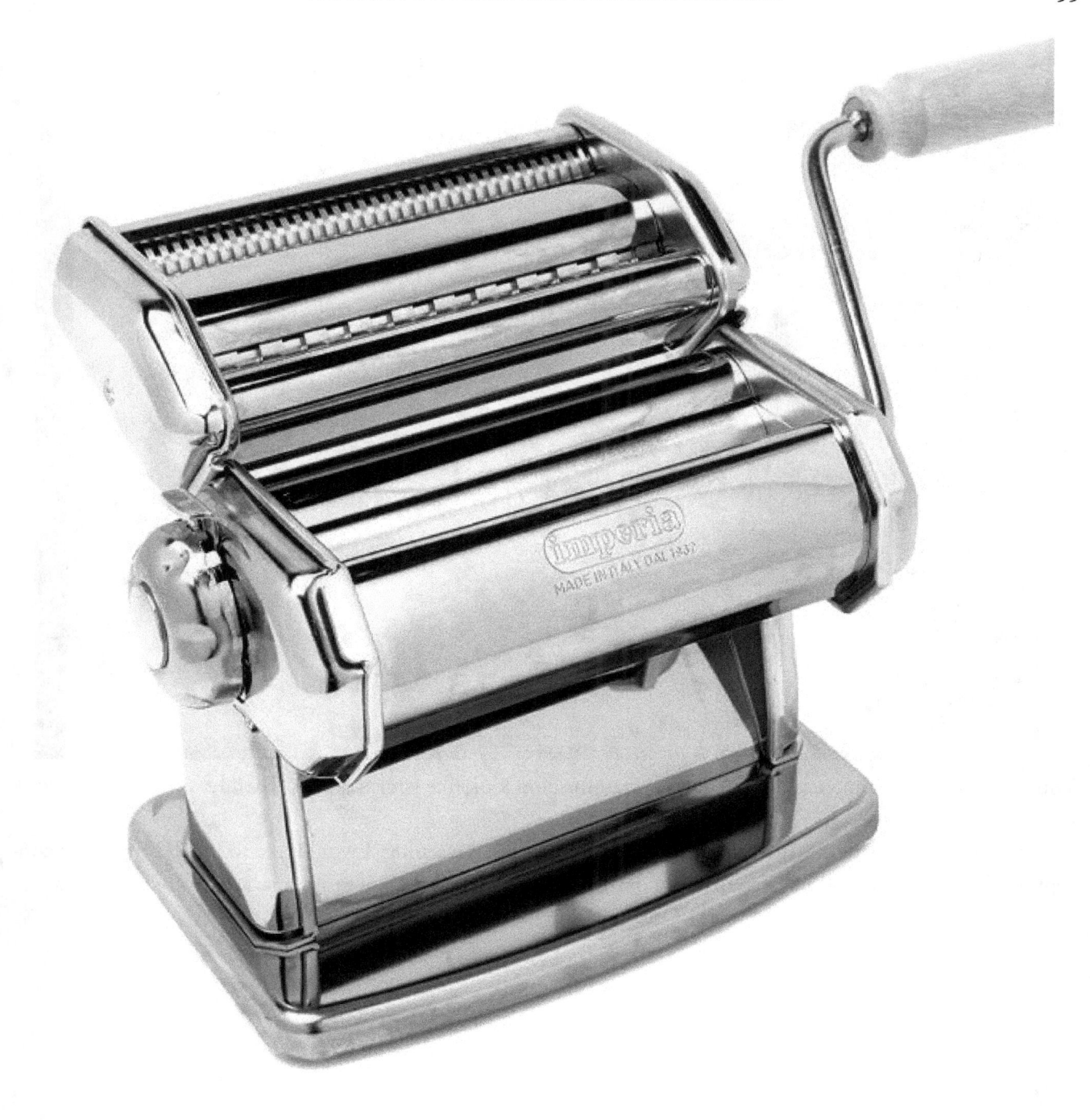

Part II - Cooking as Italians Do

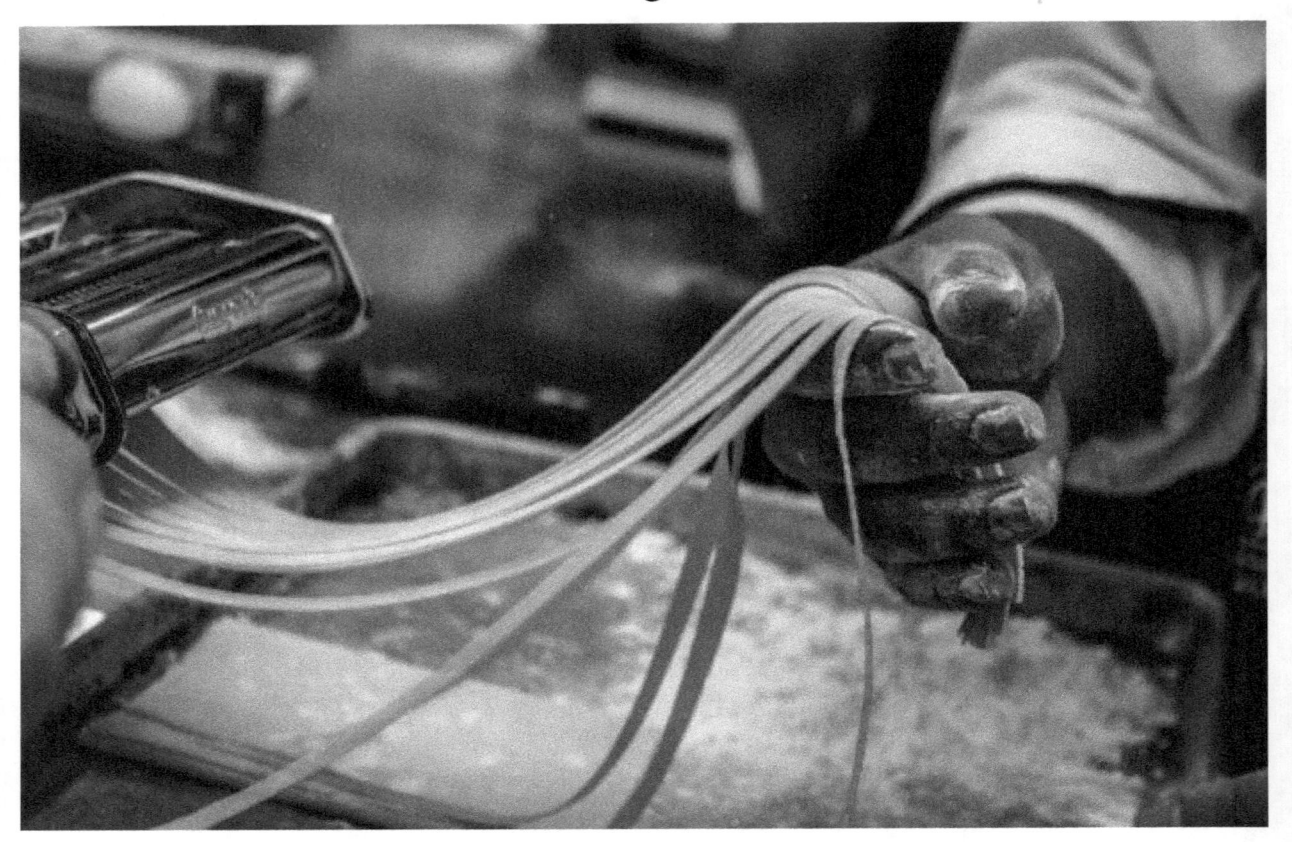

You talk like your mamma, you eat like your mamma, you look like your mamma. Then let's see if we can cook like a mamma Italiana.

In Part II we look at a little something called foundational learning. I would like to instill some clear concepts of flavor and methodology so that you don't miss a beat when it comes to preparing a full-course meal.

Chapter 5: The Foundations of Italian Cooking

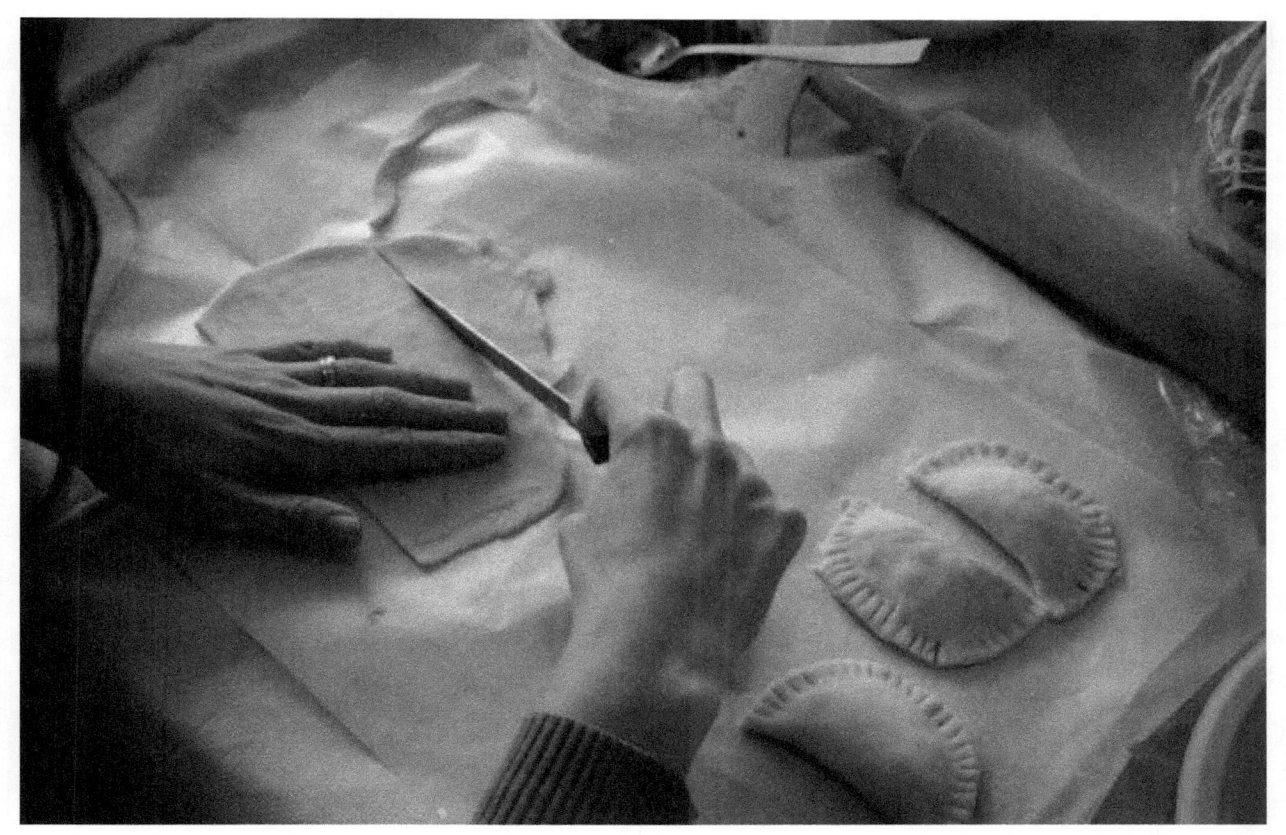

Here I have some wonderful additions to your culinary journey that will reveal a little more about the care and consideration in simplistic practices that are proven to work a charm in flavor, consistency, and ease.

You get these few things right, then the rest should follow pretty smoothly. We are experimenting, remember. Embellish in the art of learning and taking a few tries to get it 100%.

Basic Rules and Techniques

There are rules and techniques that help beginners get a solid footing. Here are some of the basics:

Odori, Battuto, and Soffritto

The preparation of fresh vegetables as a base is an important aspect of the cuisine.

Odori, which literally translates to "smells," are what we would call the infusers of most dishes. These are celery, carrots, ripe tomatoes, onions, or a pinch of basil and parsley that when added elevate the aroma and entice your sense of smell towards the meal, bringing life to any soup or broth.

The battuto is a way to prepare these odori, other than just dropping them in a pot of water, of course. A battuto requires you to chop up the odori finely (mamma would use a mezzaluna knife) together to be used in soups or added with minced meat. The finer the texture, the more flavor is imbued into the dish. There are different battuti for certain dishes, however, traditionally you should never mix onion and garlic in the same battuto.

A soffritto now is the cooking portion of this exercise. Italians love olive oil, herbs, and garlic, so you would take these minced vegetables and sauté them in olive oil, some chopped garlic, a can of tomato puree, and you have the basic foundation.

The 10 Commandments of Italian Cooking

1. <u>Keep Quality Ingredients</u>

The numero uno of all things Italian is choosing the right foundational ingredients. What comes simplest but most effective? Produce that is fresh, packs a ton of flavor, and is relatively easy to find. Go to the market to look for organic and clean vegetables, fresh cuts of meat, and fruit. Shop wisely, use beautifully.

1. <u>Use Reliable Tools and Techniques</u>

A good pan, a good knife, proper knife cuts, dressing pasta correctly, as well as kneading and cooking al dente are valuable to any aspiring cook. You want to know that what you use is reliable and will help you get the best final dish.

1. <u>Easy on the Herbs and Spices</u>

No need to over salt. Sea salt is used while cooking, in regulated amounts. Same with pepper. This is rarely added while at the table. Let the fresh natural flavor come through. Herbs are used fresh in cooking, or as a decoration when served.

1. <u>Seasonal Eating</u>

Italians use food as their main celebration of seasonal transitions. Cooking dishes with seasonal vegetables and meats is where tradition stems.

1. <u>Understanding How to Cook Pasta</u>

The art to cooking pasta comes both in timing and regular testing of the pasta itself. Are you adding a little olive oil to the water? Are you adding in a pinch of coarse salt?

1. <u>As You Cook You Taste</u>

We spoke about seasoning gently; the best way to get to know how light or heavy your hand is is by tasting.

1. <u>Mastering Your Soffritto</u>

Understanding the limitlessness of a good soffritto is crucial. It can be a last-minute prep that combines well with another meal, or a meal on its own. These sauteed vegetables need to be cooked sufficiently and adding a drop or two of wine to the soffritto to balance the flavor and elevate others is a good idea.

1. Your Sauce, Of Course

Italians focus on their base. The sauce in pasta is an addition, but be sure to not separate the pasta from the sauce; always serve them together. Also, add a little pasta water to the pot while you toss the pasta into the sauce as the starch in the water will up the flavor.

1. Easy on the Parmesan Cheese

Less is more. Cheese on pasta is a palletizing effect; add no more than 2 tsp of grated parmesan per dish.

1. Serve Your Meals Correctly

For example, risotto or pasta are never served with salads. Appetizers (starters) are served small but are very tasty. One will usually start with a vast array of antipasti or appetizers, which would consist of all kinds of vegetables and cured meats. Then the main dish of pasta is served, followed by a small dish of protein and maybe a dessert. Think of it as a reverse crescendo of flavors from the intense starter to the subtle and simple main.

Cheeses

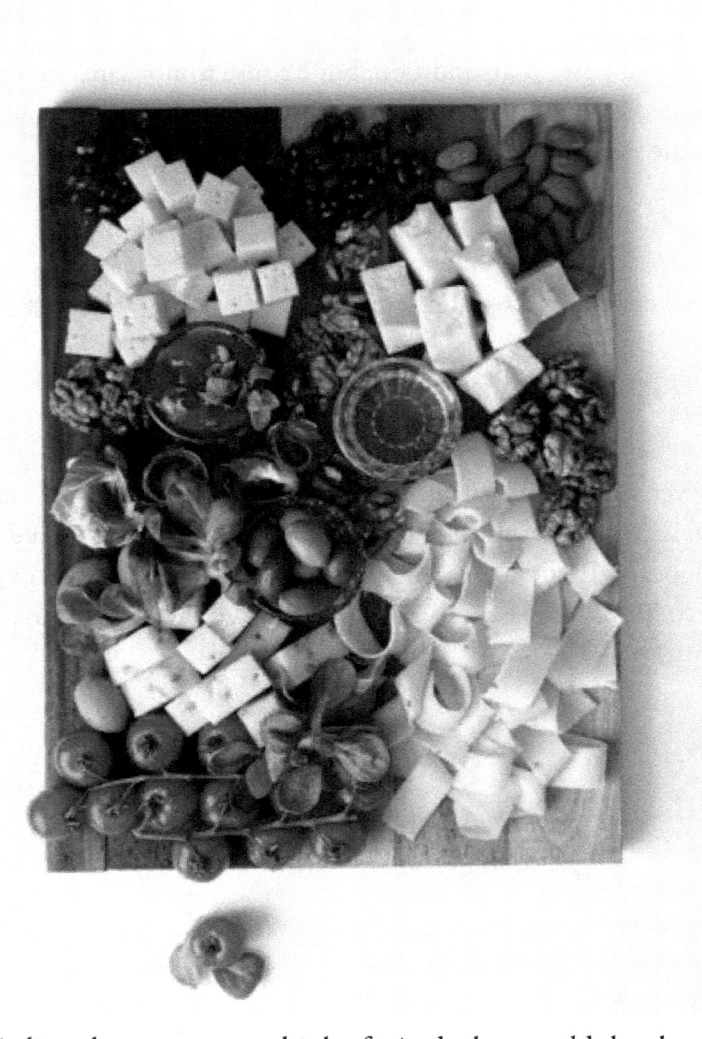

How many Italian cheeses can you think of? And what would they best be suited with?
Let's take a look:

- <u>Soft cheeses</u> like mozzarella, ricotta, mascaropen, gorgonzola, burrato, provolone, and fontina are best for thickening up meals due to their texture when heated up; they are also used in desserts as a base.

- <u>Semi-soft cheeses</u> like taleggio, asiago, and scamorza show the best of both worlds by being added into dishes or eaten fresh.

- <u>Hard cheeses</u> like parmesan, caprino, grana padano, and pecorino when grated or sliced work wonderfully in all different dishes; they are a lot stronger in taste.

Easy Peasy Ricotta at Home

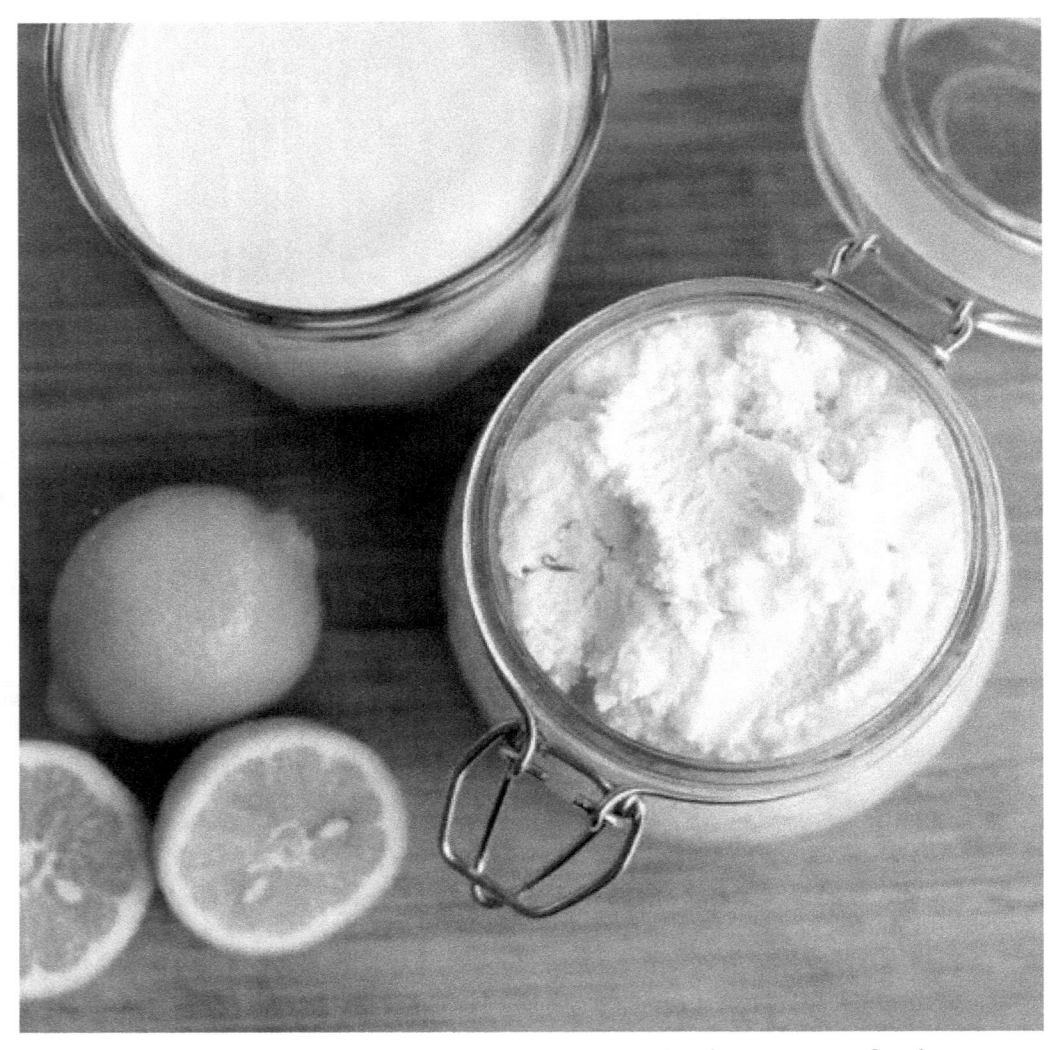

Making ricotta at home is really quite simple, and it can be done in time for dinner. Home recipes allow you to decide how you want it and for what occasion. Just make sure your <u>milk is not UHT pasteurized</u> as it might prevent separation (which is what you want).

<u>Total</u>: 90 minutes
<u>Prep Time</u>: 80 minutes (mostly waiting)
<u>Cooking Time</u>: 10 minutes
<u>Serving Size</u>: 2 cups

Ingredients	Measurements
Whole milk	9 cups
Lemon juice or white vinegar	⅓ cup
Salt	Pinch

Special Equipment:

- Cheese cloth
- Strainer
- Food thermometer
- Slotted spoon

Directions:

1. Set a large saucepan at medium heat and pour in the milk. Allow the milk to warm to 200°F by keeping an eye on your food thermometer and watch for the foam that forms. As soon as it starts to boil, take it off the plate.
2. Gently stir in your lemon juice or vinegar, while also adding the salt.
3. Now let it stand for 10 minutes so the whey (yellowish water) may separate from the curd (white floating clumps) naturally. Check the milk consistency by using the slotted spoon to shift away clumps and make sure it has all separated.
4. When you are sure you have fully separated the batch, you can now begin sifting out the curd by covering the strainer in cheesecloth tightly and placing the strainer over a bowl. Scoop out the largest clumps first and then pour the remaining whey through the strainer.
5. Take the cheesecloth strainer and let it sit for around 1 hour to drain. The longer you wait, the more dry it will be.
6. Use the cheesecloth as a pressure device to squeeze out the remaining moisture and then place spoonfuls of the ricotta in the glass jars for storage or later use.

Nifty Tips:

- If your milk doesn't curdle, just add a little more lemon juice and wait a tad longer to see it seperate.

- Do not throw away that lovely whey that you have collected. It has the right acidic content to be used in sauces and baking the next day.

Pasta

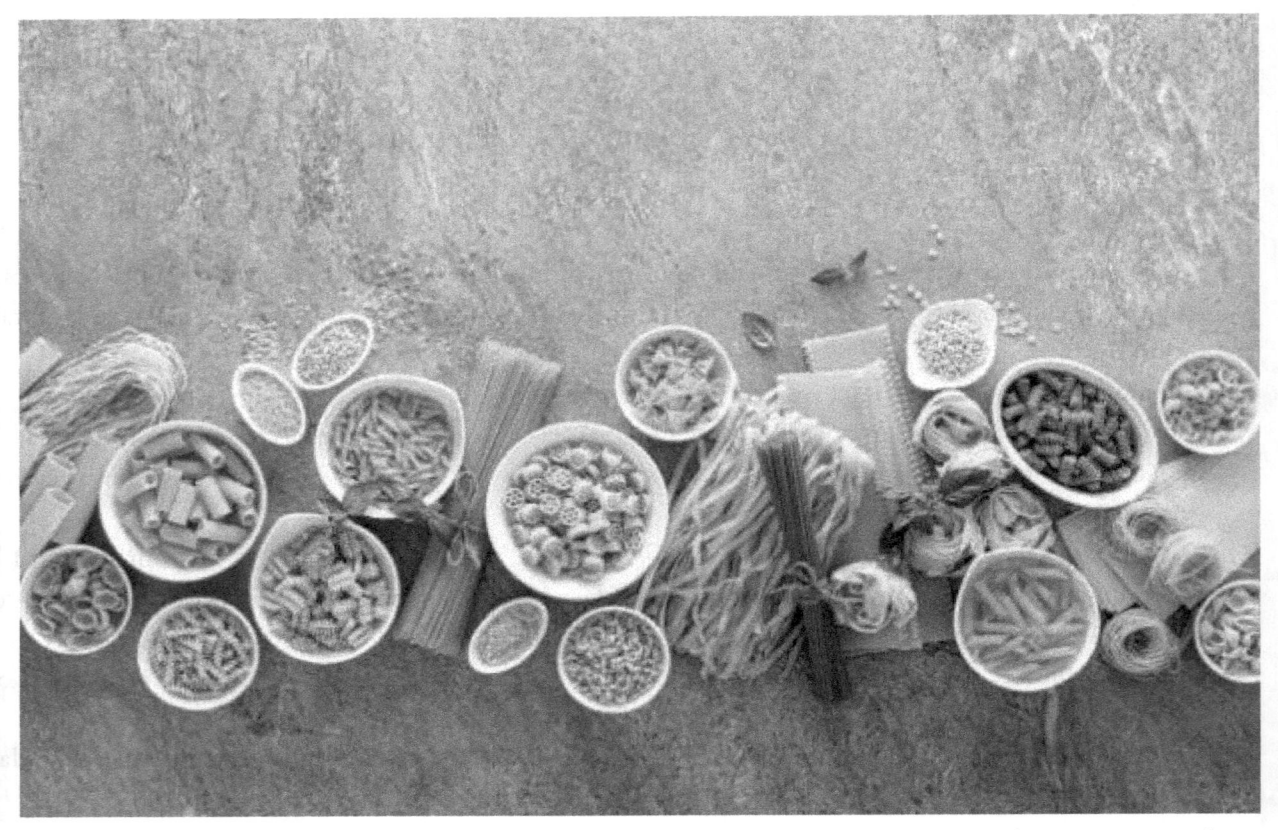

What types do we have to choose from? Plenty! The question is, what are you going to be serving it with? Each pasta is best suited both in tradition and in practicality to certain sauces and proteins. Let's take a look:

- Strand pasta is a lengthy string of pasta that we commonly see as spaghetti, bigoli, capellini, vermicelli, or picini. It is best used in a light sauce, with tomato and garlic.

- Shaped pasta includes fusilli, orecchiette, conchiglie, casarecce, rotini, caratelle, farfalle, gemelli, and campanelle. These are best used in very rich sauces that can balance the larger shapes of pasta.

- Ribbon pasta is also lengthy but with a wider shape like lasagna, linguine, tagliatelle, tagliolini, pappardelle, and mafaldine. These are best used in rich sauces with heavy cream and cheese.

- Soup pasta is small delicate pasta swimming in a soup or broth like orzo and ditalini. It's best used in light soups and broths.

- Tubular pasta are hollow and include bucatini, penne, rigatoni, macaroni, paccheri, cannelloni, and manicotti. These are best used in thin sauces that can flow into the center with strong aromatic flavors.

- <u>Stuffed pasta</u> is softer pasta like mezzalune, ravioli, tortellini, mautasche, and cappelletti. They are best used in broths and are filled with light cheeses, herbs, and delicate meats.

- <u>Gnocchi</u> is not technically a pasta, although this traditional potato dumpling is as much a staple as pasta itself. It's best served with meaty and rich sauces that balance the dense and chewy bite-sized gnocchi.

The Principles

1. The three principles of making pasta are flour, eggs, and time. The flour is your base, and the eggs bring in the moisture and fat content. One could use egg yolks alone or egg whites alone. I would not recommend making homemade pasta with just water. Sometimes a recipe will call for adding a little oil to the mix to help the egg mix in well with the flour and allow that gluten to develop.
2. Stuffed or filled pasta needs to only be used with 00 pasta and semolina and the filling needs to be dry and compact before insertion. The pasta goes in with gently boiling water. Once they float, they are cooked. Strand, shaped, and ribbon pasta works better with the semolina. Sometimes halving semolina and 00 pasta into a recipe can bring all the components of each into a pasta to make it hardier and tastier. That is why you would find that 00 pasta is best suited for an egg recipe, and semolina is more suitable for a white pasta (or hardier pasta) recipe.
3. What is the biggest difference between fresh and store-bought dried pasta you ask? It boils down to (excuse the pun) the texture, flavor, and use. Home-made fresh pasta has a substantial fluffiness and wholesome gusto that you cannot find in dried options. The reason behind this is the use of eggs and flour in the dough that keeps the flavor sealed but will not last if stored. Dried pasta contains only semolina flour and water which allow it to be stored for longer periods.
4. Never put pasta in when the water is boiling hard. Rather, just wait for the water to fully boil, then lower the heat slightly. The worst you can do is overcook the pasta! Al dente is the best way to go, meaning that when the pasta comes out of the water, it can still cook a little when it is placed in the hot sauce. Always add in a pinch of coarse salt and a drizzle of olive oil to your water before you drop in your pasta.
5. If you keep quality pasta or make it yourself, then you will not need exaggerated sauces or excessive cheese to make the meal delicious. The pasta itself is the main meal, the rest is the garnish. Learning to appreciate and savor good pasta (and good bread, which we touch on soon) is what I want you to do. Toppings also do not have to be extraordinary, just simple, fresh, and cooked with love.
6. Dried pasta needs to be boiled for much longer than fresh pasta.
7. The dough must be elastic but not crumbly. It should leave your hands dry and not sticky. Too wet can bring about breakage.
8. What about colored pasta? Green pasta can be made by adding boiled spinach water, black pasta needs squid ink powder, and red pasta uses boiled beetroot water. Or just use food colorants.

Make Pasta at Home Like Mamma

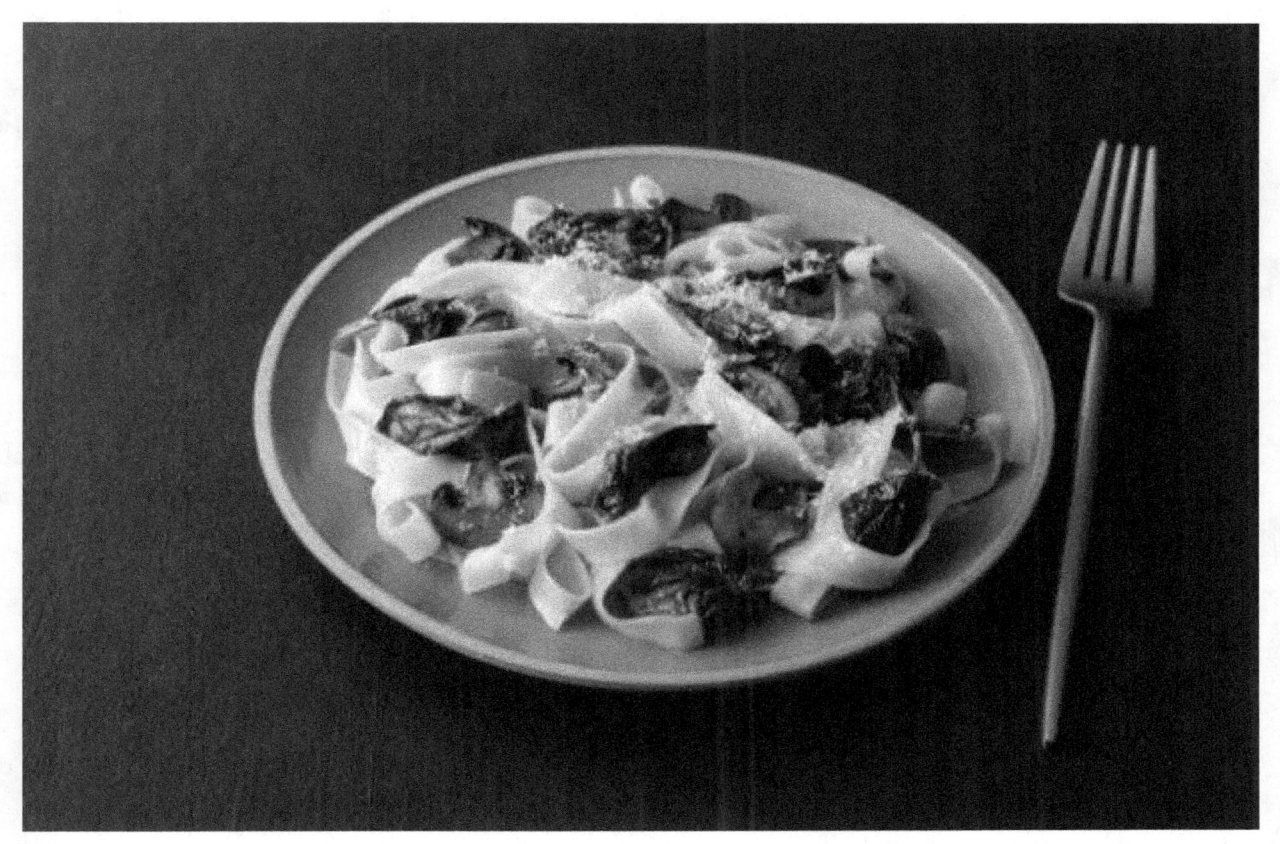

Here is a basic soft and fluffy pasta dough recipe that will get you working with your hands and marveling at your final product.

If you have a stable surface, two hands, some flour, eggs, and a roller, you can make pasta!

This recipe (technically a method on its own) will be split into two different practices of rolling your pasta. The first is the easy machine method and the second is a more rigorous hand method.

Total Time: 1 hour 20 minutes (includes rising)

Ingredients Measurements

AP flour   2 cups
Eggs   2
Salt   1 tsp

Special Equipment:

- Rolling pin
- Bench scraper
- Pasta machine (both flat and teeth attachments needed)

Directions:

1. Begin by shaking out the flour onto your clean surface and making a small well in the middle of the flour.
2. Break the 2 eggs into the well, add your salt, and begin mixing the egg into the flour gently with a fork as if you were scrambling them up. Some prefer to add in a touch of olive oil, but it should not be necessary if you have the eggs.
3. Once the flour and egg in the middle of the well have been combined, take your bench scraper and begin scraping all the loose bits into the center while combining with the other hand. The surface should be relatively clean around the dough before you begin kneading. If too dry, spray *a little* water over the surface and keep kneading. If too wet, sprinkle some flour instead.
4. Kneading dough should feel like a periodic movement of the wrist. You push with the heel of your palm and pull back towards yourself with your fingers so as to incorporate the flour evenly into the eggs. 10 minutes should do the trick. Once the dough is smooth and elastic (you have created a stable gluten network) then it is ready to rest. Wrap the dough ball in plastic and place it somewhere cool for around an hour so it can build more moisture and relax.

Now if you have a machine, that's great! Follow as below:

1. Cut your dough ball into equal segments with your bench scraper or knife, working with each segment separately to make the process more manageable.
2. Using your rolling pin, roll out a segment to around 1-inch thickness making sure that the shape of the dough is even and will fit the attachment to your machine.
3. The roller attachments will allow you to quickly and effortlessly lengthen and reduce the thickness of the pasta. You will allow the dough to pass through the roller once, then fold it into itself twice (laminating), and then feed it through the roller two more times while laminating and keeping a rectangle shape to the dough.
4. Depending on the type of pasta you are making, for instance, fettuccine or ravioli, then the thickness will have to be determined by adjusting the width of the rollers in the machine (thin enough to be able to slightly see your fingers through the dough). Make sure to always have the widest setting in your rollers to prevent crimping.
5. Eventually, you will have long thin dough that is ready to be cut and placed on a clean towel with some flour sprinkled over so it does not sweat and stick together.
6. Put that sheet aside and repeat the process with the other segments of dough.

Making pasta without a machine can seem daunting, but let's just take a quick look at how this can work:

1. Sprinkle some flour onto your clean surface and place your dough segment down for manual rolling.
2. When rolling out your dough by hand you want to keep the same strategy as the above method with the machine, meaning that you will roll out and then laminate the dough three times as well.

3. Once laminating is complete, we want to get that dough into a thinner rectangle. If the dough keeps on retracting as you roll it out then just wait for a second or two for the gluten to relax and then keep rolling it out from there. Just like above, we want to be able to see our fingers ever so slightly through the surface.
4. From there, we can cut the sheet into whatever shape needed, and place it aside on a floured surface to rest while you move onto the next segment.

Bread Basics

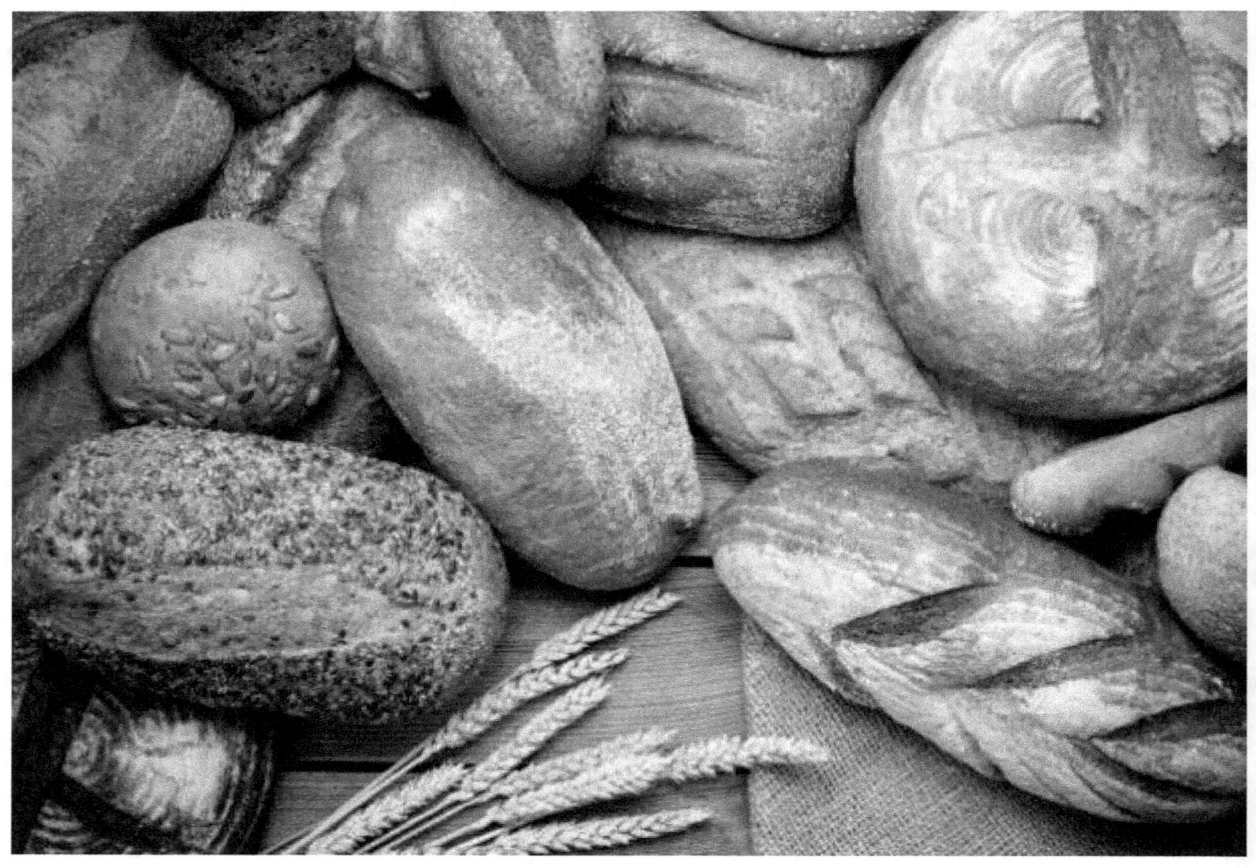

The delicious crumbly texture of a fresh-baked bread. Oh my! Nothing competes.

Pane (bread) is vital at the Italian table. Bread is rarely brought to the table in a basket, but rather placed directly on the tablecloth to be pinched and shared throughout the meal. If there are crumbs all over the tablecloth, you have done a good job!

So what exactly are the bread basics? As it goes, Italians are pretty particular about what gets put on their tables. You could call it a prideful choice. And of course, if you have some pieces hanging around that need to be eaten, be sure to see Nonno (grandad) dunking that last piece into his red wine, saying "*Gli da gusto!*", or "It gives taste!".

Here are some of the most common bread out there that are never amiss on an Italian table:

- Ciabatta
- Coppia Ferrese
- Ciriola
- Focaccia
- Pugliese

- Altopascio
- Certosino
- Ciambella
- Toscano

Some can be found at your local supermarket, while others require a bit of sniffing around for an artisan baker to get the right quality. But what if you want to make your own? I'll take you through a recipe for basic bread that can be infused and one for soft delicious focaccia.

Bread is made with four standard ingredients: flour, water, salt, and yeast. All-purpose flour works just fine to start out, although purchasing bread flour can create a denser and chewy texture due to the protein content.

So how do you get that typical crunchy crust and super soft interior? In technicality, it is all about the moisture (steam) at the beginning of the baking process. Spraying water before and 5 minutes into the bake can allow the bread to form a crust. One could also brush egg wash (1 egg mixed with a little water) onto the surface of the dough or alternatively boil water in a skillet in the oven to create steam for the dough to draw in and expand. Then remove the skillet after 5 minutes so the bread may bake and crust.

Instant yeast does not require proofing, while active yeast does. So keep that in mind when deciding which to use.

To check if you have kneaded your dough sufficiently, you can just poke the surface with your finger, and if the dough bounces back quickly, then it is ready to be popped into the oven to bake.

Greasing the inside of the bowl and the surface of the dough before the rising and proofing stages assists in retaining moisture and flavor. If you are feeling adventurous, you could easily add diverse flavors like rosemary or pitted olives (or both!) into the dough before baking.

In terms of trays, you could use standard baking sheets or a bread bin. Italian bread needs to be a typical shape and crust, therefore on a sheet is preferred.

Italian Bread at Home

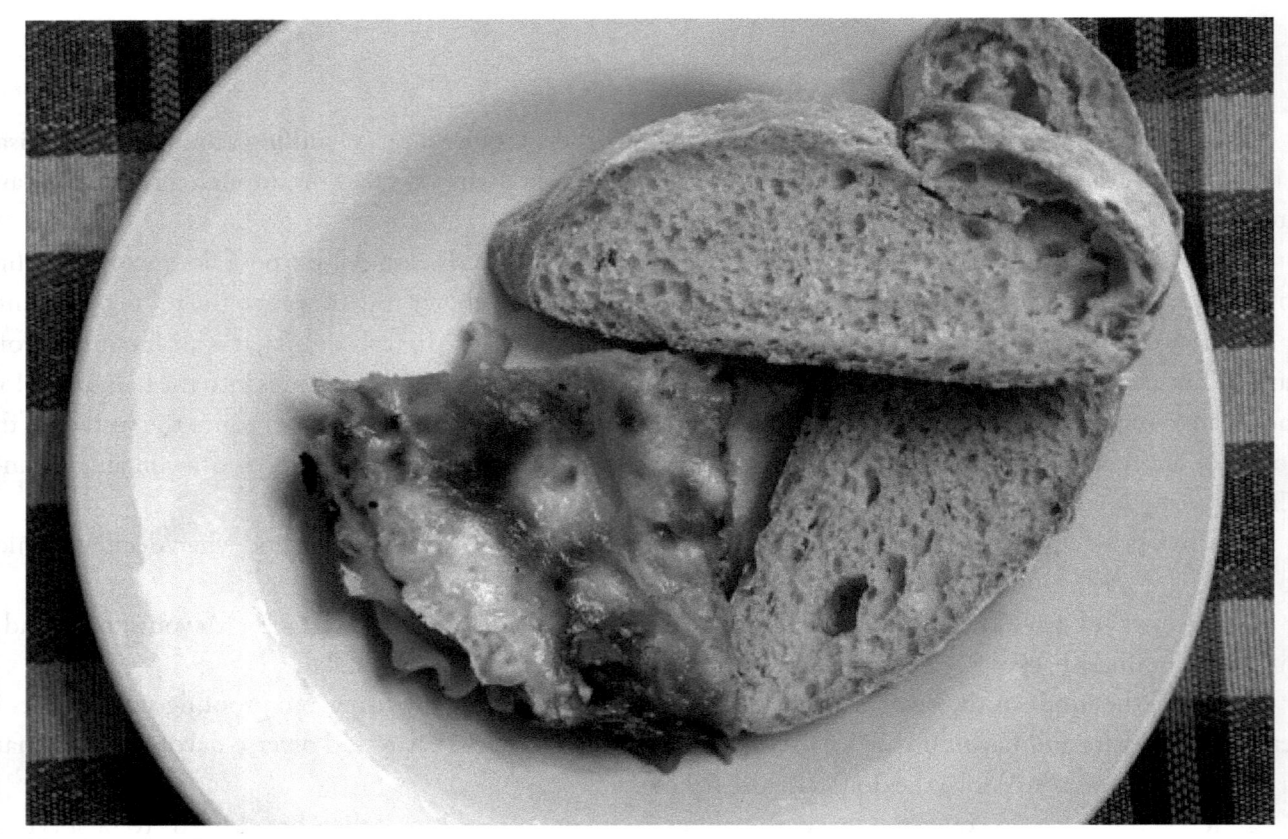

<u>Total</u>: 2 hours and 20 minutes
<u>Prep Time</u>: 1 hour and 50 minutes (includes rising and proofing)
<u>Baking Time</u>: 30 minutes
<u>Serving Size</u>: 2 loaves

Ingredients	Measurements
AP flour	5 cups
Warm water (100 °F / 38 °C)	2 cups
Salt	2 tsp
Sugar	1 tsp
Instant yeast	1 sachet

<u>Special Equipment</u>:

- Standing mixer with bread paddle attachment

<u>Directions</u>:

1. Begin by inserting the following into your mixer: 2 cups of flour, salt, sugar, yeast, and warm water. Let the paddle do its thing on a medium speed until you can see that all the flour is mixed in properly.
2. The mixture should be quite stodgy; add in the remaining 3 cups of flour slowly to ensure that you get the right consistency (sticking to the paddle).
3. Spoon out the dough and place it on a floured surface so that you may begin the kneading process. Knead for 10 minutes and add a tad more flour or a spray of water to make sure that the dough is not too dry or too wet. Smooth and tacky is great.
4. In a large bowl, place the dough ball and cover it with plastic wrap. Place the bowl in a warm area to rise for approximately 1 hour.
5. Divide the risen dough into two segments and shape them into logs on a floured surface. It helps to pinch the corners to allow the dough to rise in a more precise shape.
6. Place the logs on a baking tray and line them with baking paper. Cover again with plastic wrap and place in a warm area for a further 30 minutes. This is a good time to start preheating your oven to 400 °F (205 °C).
7. Remove the plastic wrap and score the surface of the dough with a knife to allow the bread to expand in a preferred shape. Then, place it in the oven for around 30 minutes to bake, noticing it turn a golden brown.
8. Allow the bread to cool for around 10 minutes before serving.

Focaccia Done Well

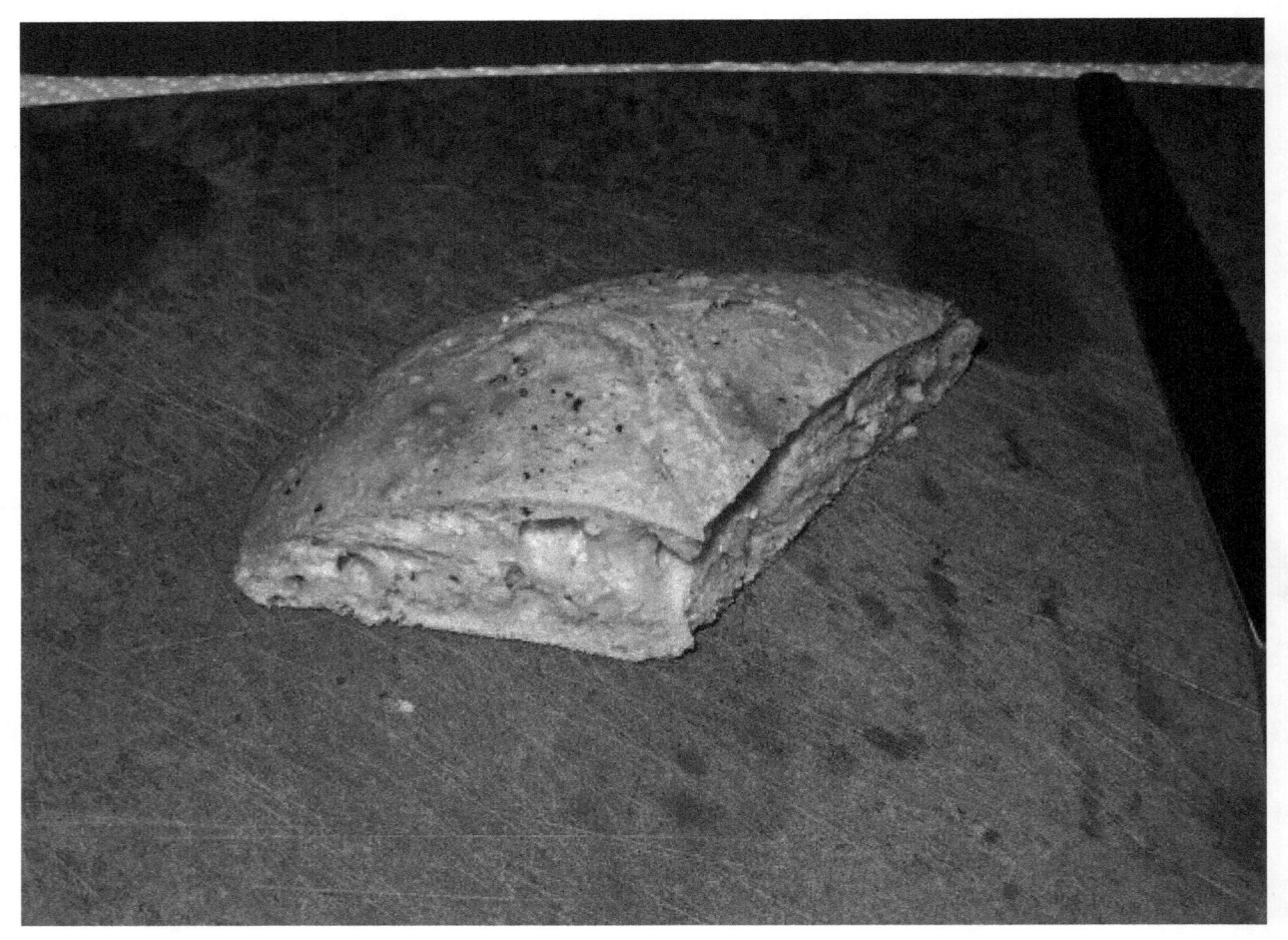

With focaccia bread, we tend to see more yeast, olive oil, and salt in the mix, as well as a longer proofing stage. The texture of focaccia needs to be fluffy and light, oily and flavorful. Again, AP flour works well, but consider trying bread flour to assert your taste buds.

It can be super useful to think about getting baking steel or baking ceramic tiles that you place in the oven before you bake. This is especially true with focaccia that needs consistent heat.

Total: 1 hour
Prep Time: 30 minutes
Baking Time: 30 minutes
Serving Size: 6 to 8 servings

Ingredients	Measurements
AP flour	3 ¼ cups
Lukewarm water (68 °F / 20 °C)	1 ½ cup + 3 tbsp
Olive oil	5 tbsp
Instant dry yeast	½ sachet
Coarse salt	1 tbsp
Table salt	2 tsp

Special Equipment:

- Standing mixer with whisk attachment
- Skillet (12 inches)
- Dough scraper
- Baking steel

Directions:

1. Begin by inserting the following into your mixer: flour, salt, yeast, and warm water. Whisk until the mixture is uniform and transfer to a large bowl. If it looks dry add one tablespoon of water at a time mixing manually to get a moist but not sticky ball of dough.
2. Add 1 ½ tbsp of olive oil and use your hands to mix it into the dough. Cover the bowl with plastic wrap and let it rest for around 1 hour at room temperature.
3. After removing the plastic wrap, take your dough scraper and fold the dough into itself six times by lifting the edges towards the center and alternating sides at each fold. Then cover with the wrap again and allow it to rest another 15 minutes.
4. The same folding process is repeated once more, then covered again, and placed in the refrigerator for 18 hours to 3 days (the longer the better).
5. When you believe that your dough has rested long enough, let the bowl return to room temperature for around 10 minutes before placing it on a floured surface.
6. Flour your hands well and begin shaping the dough into a rounded ball by folding the edges inwards and underneath, creating a seam at the bottom.
7. Cover the bottom of your skillet with 2 tbsp of olive oil. Place the dough in the skillet, turn it in the oil and then flatten the dough to fill the skillet base evenly. Once again, we will cover the surface with plastic wrap and allow it to rest for 2 hours at room temperature.
8. An hour before baking, you will preheat the oven to 500°F (260 °C) and insert the baking steel on a middle rack. You can take the skillet and lift the edges of the dough ever so gently around the circumference to release air bubbles. Use your finger to lightly indent the dough (dimpling) then brush the surface with 1 ½ tbsp of olive oil and the coarse salt.
9. It's finally baking time! Place the skillet on top of the baking steel. Around 15 minutes into the bake, rotate the skillet to even out the golden-brown surface. Leave for a further 15 minutes. When the

bottom of the focaccia is also browned, then you can remove it from the oven.
10. Transfer to a drying rack, brush some olive oil over the surface and let it cool for around 5 minutes before serving.

Pizza Dough

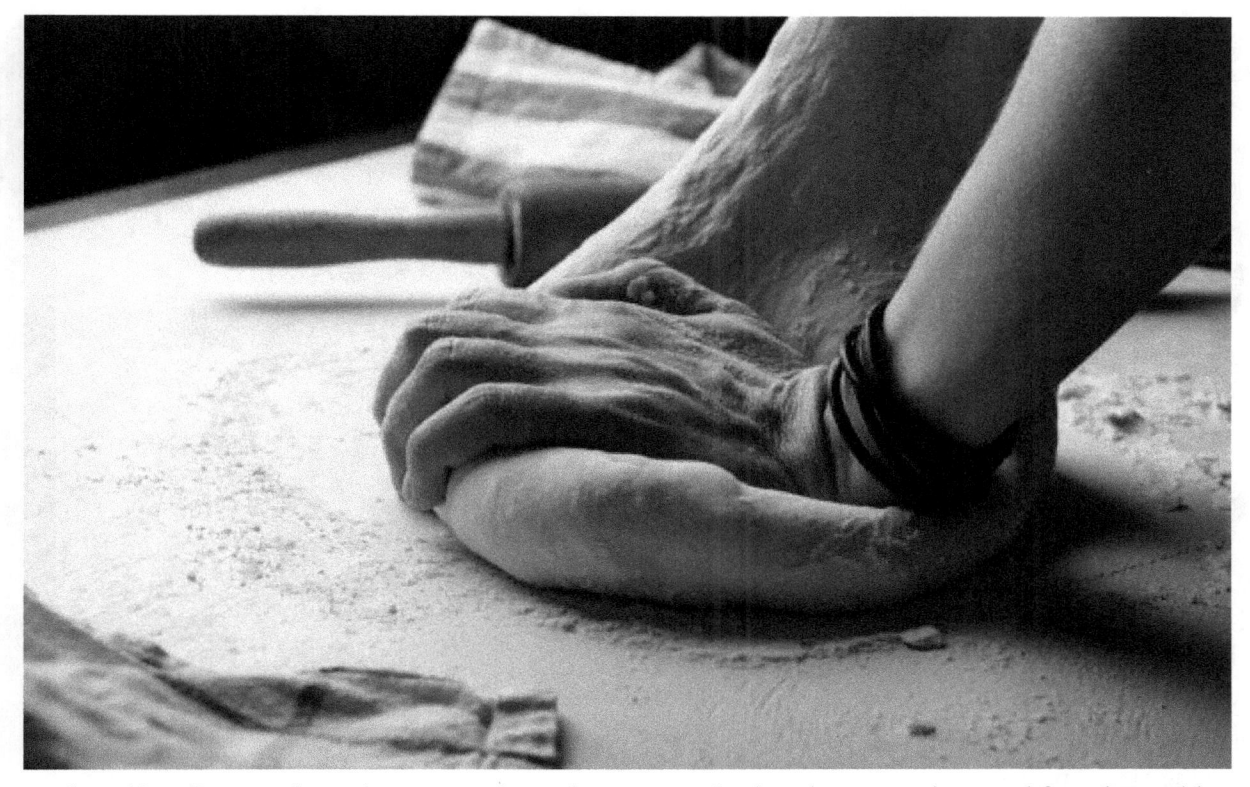

Pizza is loved by all, versatile, and easy to make and to eat. No doubt it begins with a good foundation like everything else in this cuisine.

Making pizza dough is not as challenging as you might think, but it requires some practice to get perfect. The challenge is finding the right toppings to finish off your perfect crust and turn the pizza from mediocre to absolutely brilliant.

First things first, let's get one thing straight: pizza needs a tomato base and mozzarella cheese. I have seen all sorts of strange and wonderful combinations, but if you want to make a proper Italian pizza, then you do not skip these two main ingredients. You can spice up the tomato base by adding in various herbs and spices, and you can zhuzh up the cheese by buying the best quality.

After that, we can start getting a little more creative, but we should keep the toppings sparse, not overcrowded. You still want to be able to pick the pizza with your hands without all the toppings falling on your lap. So, be delicate on your placement and lighten your hand when it comes to meat.

Also, try to use more fresh herbs with your pizza, like rocket, basil, and chives. These kick the flavor up a notch and really work well with the gooey and warm cheese.

A Basic Dough

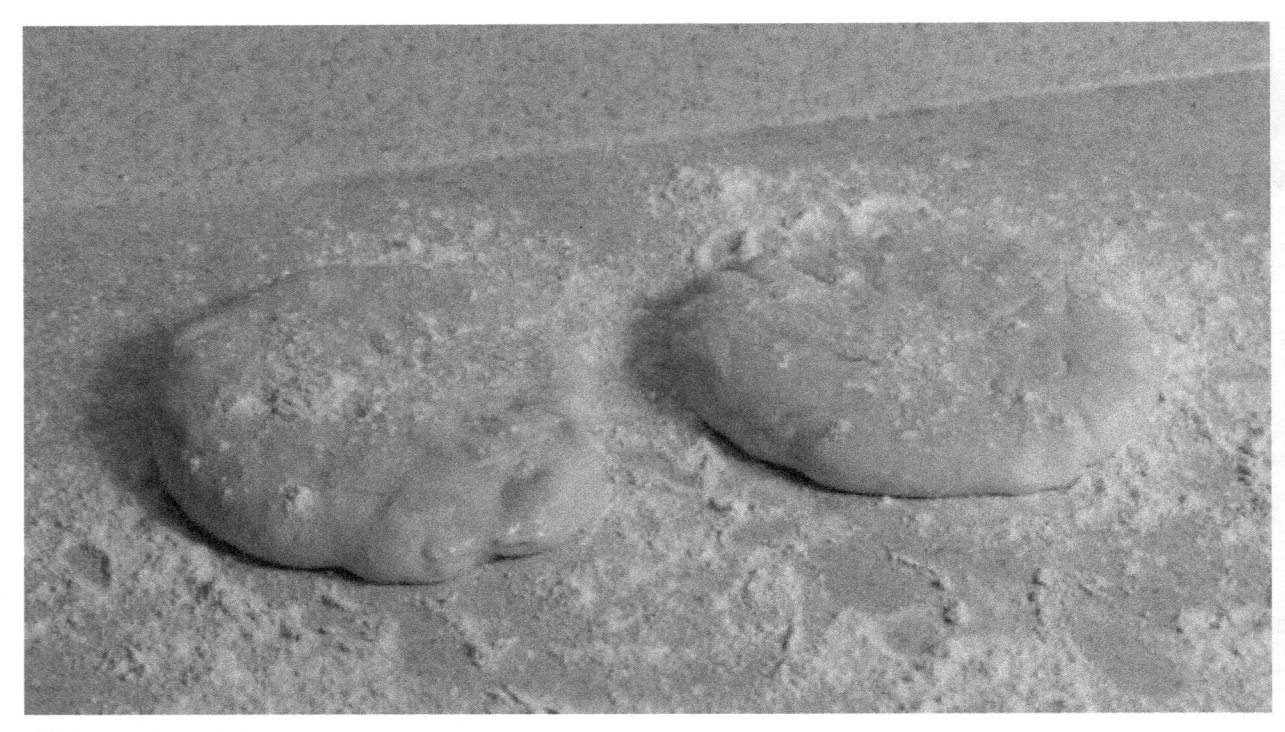

Total Time: 1 hour 30 minutes
Serving Size: 2 pizzas

Ingredients Measurements

Bread flour   4 cups
warm water   1 ½ cups
Instant yeast 1 sachet
Olive oil   3 tbsp
Salt   2 tsp
Sugar   1 tsp

Special Equipment:

- Food processor

Directions:

1. In your food processor, combine the flour, yeast, sugar, and salt. As the mixer goes, slowly pour in 2 tbsp of olive oil and the warm water. You should be left with a soft but firm ball to work with.
2. On a floured surface, knead the dough for around 10 minutes until smooth and elastic. In a greased bowl, place the kneaded dough and cover, leaving it to rise for around 1 hour.

3. Once rested, divide the dough into two sections, and return them to separate bowls to rise again for a further 10 minutes before rolling out.

<u>Nifty Tips</u>:

- If the dough is too dry, add some water, and if too wet, a sprinkle of flour.

Sauces

Making the perfect pasta sauce is an art. It might take you a few times to get the method right and understand when to add more of this and that to adjust the flavor to your liking and you will learn what each ingredient does for the dish. Once you get the knack for the methods, you will see why it is so important.

The time spent simmering directly equates to how saucy and rich the final product will be. Traditionally, sauces should cook overnight, but I suppose we are time-conscious creatures, so let us have a look at two of the most basic sauces to add to your pasta that you can start in the afternoon and have ready for your dinner.

The Tomato Sauce

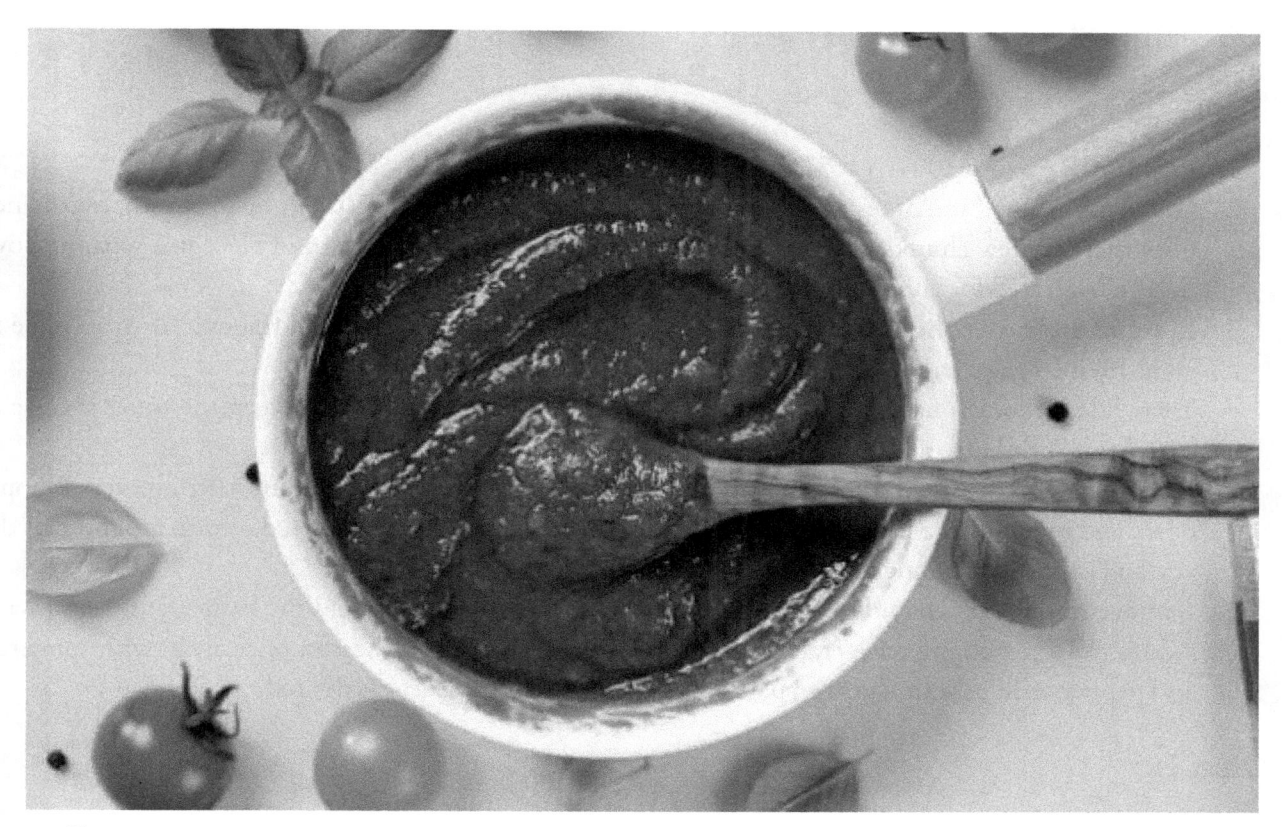

<u>Time</u>: 6 hours 10 minutes
   <u>Prep Time</u>: 10 minutes
   <u>Cooking Time</u>: 6 hours
   <u>Serving Size</u>: 8 servings

Ingredients	Measurements
Whole peeled tomatoes	28 oz (4 cans)
Carrots	1
Onion	1
Fresh basil	½ cup
Fresh parsley	1 sprig
Dried oregano	1 tbsp
Red pepper flakes	1 tsp
Garlic	8 cloves
Butter	4 tbsp
Olive oil	¼ cup
Salt and pepper	pinch

Special Equipment:

- Dutch oven

Directions:

1. Preheat the oven to 300 °F (165 °C).
2. Grab your canned tomatoes and pour them into a large bowl. Squish the tomatoes with your hands until there are few chunks in the sauce. Take around 3 cups of that sauce and place in a separate bowl to be refrigerated for later.
3. In your Dutch oven, heat up the butter and add in your minced garlic until fragrant, then sprinkle in your dried oregano and red pepper flakes. Stir for 2 minutes at high heat.
4. Then, add in your roughly chopped carrot, halved onion, basil leaves, and keep the tomato sauce at high heat. Sprinkle in a little salt and pepper.
5. Place the lid ajar on the Dutch oven and pop the sauce in the oven for 6 hours, stirring every 2 hours or so, and reducing the heat ever so slightly as you go. The sauce should be reduced to around half the size and changed to a much darker red color.
6. Remove from the oven and retrieve the onion halves, the carrot bits, and the basil stems if necessary. Add in your remaining refrigerated tomato sauce and olive oil, and season once again with some salt and pepper. Add in your chopped parsley, and serve with your pasta as desired.

Nifty Tips:

- This sauce can be frozen for 6 months.

- Remember, tomato sauce is only as good as the tomatoes you use, so try your best to purchase top-quality canned goods.

The Original Ragu

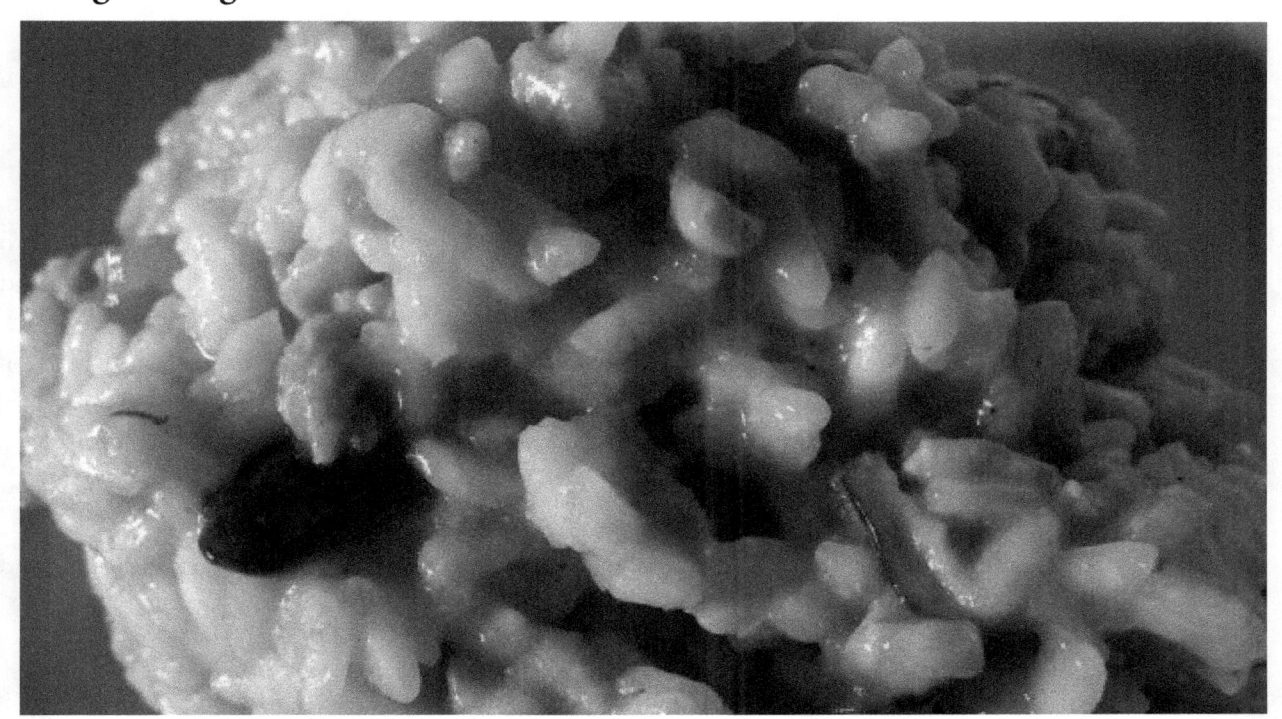

Time: 3 hours 45 minutes
　Prep Time: 10 minutes
　Cooking Time: 3 hours 35 minutes
　Serving Size: 16 servings

Ingredients	Measurements
Homemade broth	2 cups
Ground beef	4 lb
Carrots	2
Onions	2
Celery	3 ribs
Tomato paste	¼ cup
Unsalted butter	3 tbsp
Powder gelatin	2 sachets
Bay leaves	2
White or red wine	1 ½ cups
Heavy cream	½ cup
Fish sauce	½ tsp
Nutmeg	pinch
Salt and pepper	pinch

Special Equipment:

- Dutch oven

Directions:

1. In a bowl, add in your broth and sprinkle over the gelatin, then set aside for later use.
2. In your Dutch oven, heat up the butter to medium-high heat until lightly foaming. Now, add in your finely minced carrots, celery, and onions until they are soft and glassy, which should be around 6 minutes.
3. Now we can add in the ground beef, stirring for 15 minutes to break up the contents and cook evenly.
4. Lower the heat and add in your tomato paste; pour in your wine, and bring to a slow boil. Allow the wine to evaporate for 5 minutes before adding in your bay leaves.
5. Next we pour in the broth, sprinkle it with nutmeg, salt, pepper, and let it gently simmer for 3 hours. Then you can remove the bay leaves and skim some of the excess fat off the surface.
6. Season with a little more salt and pepper and add in your heavy cream. Stir for 5 more minutes and it is ready to serve with your pasta of choice.

Nifty Tips:

- You could very well increase the flavor by using half beef mince and half pork mince for meat.

- You can decide how rich you would like the ragú to be by either using a subtle vegetable broth or stronger meat broth.

Part III - 50 Italian Delicacies Just For You

ITALIAN COOKBOOK FOR EVERYDAY USE. 89

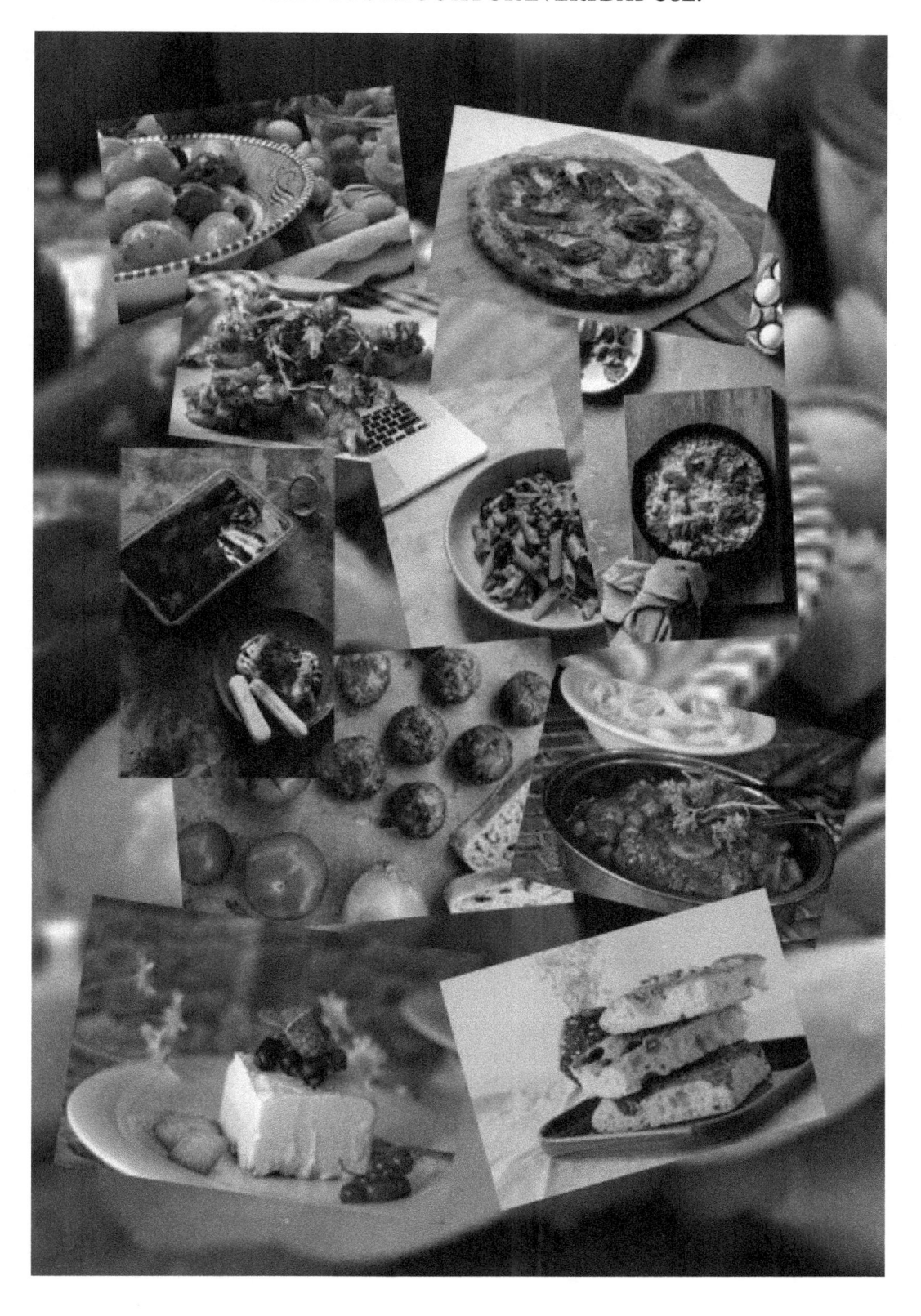

Now comes the good part! Let us devour some of the most common and popular Italian dishes that are out there.

In Part III we will be looking at some beautiful and simple starters, then touching on cheeses, soups, a little risotto, some polenta, and of course, pasta and pizza. Let us not forget the salads and the desserts.

Some are quick and simple, and some need a little more concentration, but they are doable and entirely within your reach if you are willing to try.

Chapter 6: Antipasti [Appetizers]

Like any live performance, there is always a time to set the stage or theme and to invigorate the audience and get them excited about the next performance to come. That is where we see the role of antipasti in a meal. The term *antipasto* literally translates to "before the meal."

We look at the colors, the smell, and the freshness of the starter. They can be raw or cooked. The majority of these dishes can be served quickly and effortlessly, with beautiful and sometimes hidden flavor combinations.

These were traditionally set in place to bring about more appetite and introduce the rest of the meal as a starter performance, as an appetite increaser, or simply as a small meal to have while the guests wait for their main course.

The point is, this starter needs to be compelling. It can be simple but unique and invigorating.

Marinated Olives

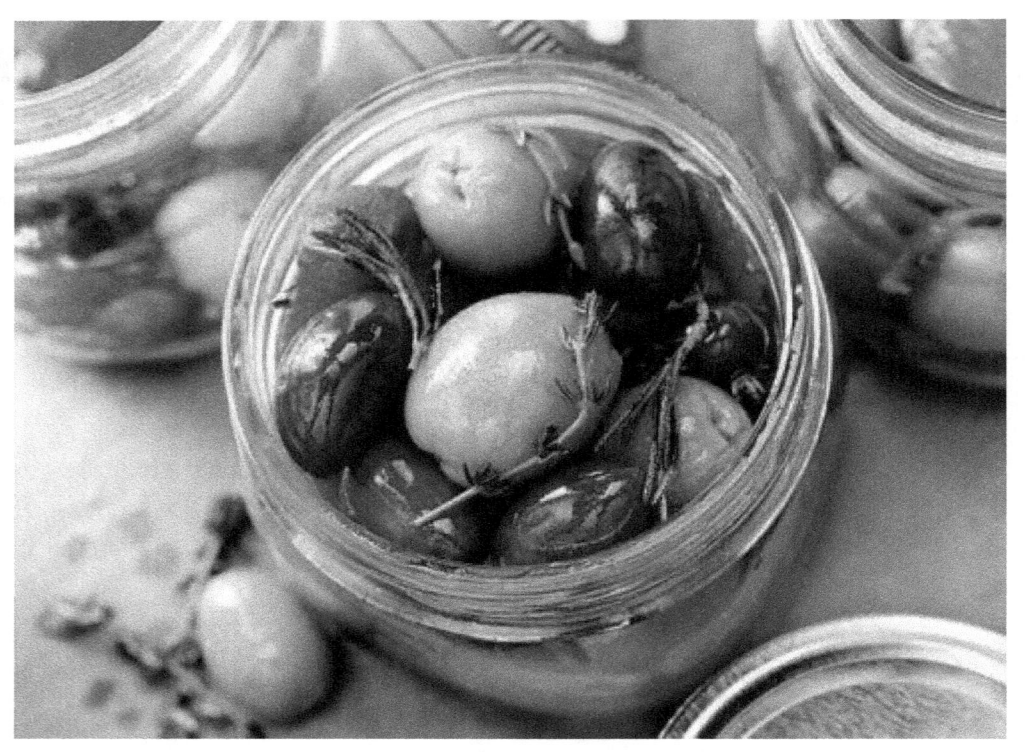

On the table you will see a bowl of olives, delicately placed, oily and savory, with a toothpick holder close by. It's the perfect starter to allow you to get your stomach rumbling and happy vibes flowing around the table.

Total Prep Time: 10 minutes

Serving Size: 6 to 8 servings

Ingredients	Measurements
Unpitted olives	1 ⅜ cups
Olive oil	3 tbsp
Fennel seeds	½ tbsp
Fresh parsley	Small handful
Dried oregano	1 tsp
Garlic	½ clove
Chili or red pepper flakes	1 tsp
Lemon	1
Pepper	Pinch

Directions:

1. Grab a large bowl and place within it the fennel seeds, oregano, minced garlic, chili flakes, lemon zest,

and pepper. Mix it all up well and allow it to rest for a couple of minutes.
2. Next you will finely dice up the parsley and add it along with the olive oil into the bowl.
3. Drain the olives to remove the taste of brine, then place them in the bowl, toss them with vigor and let that rest for another couple of minutes before serving.

Nifty Tips:

- Unpitted olives have far more flavor and meatiness than pitted choices, although you can select other varieties if you wish.

Mozzarella Bocconcini, Pesto, and Sun Blushed Tomatoes

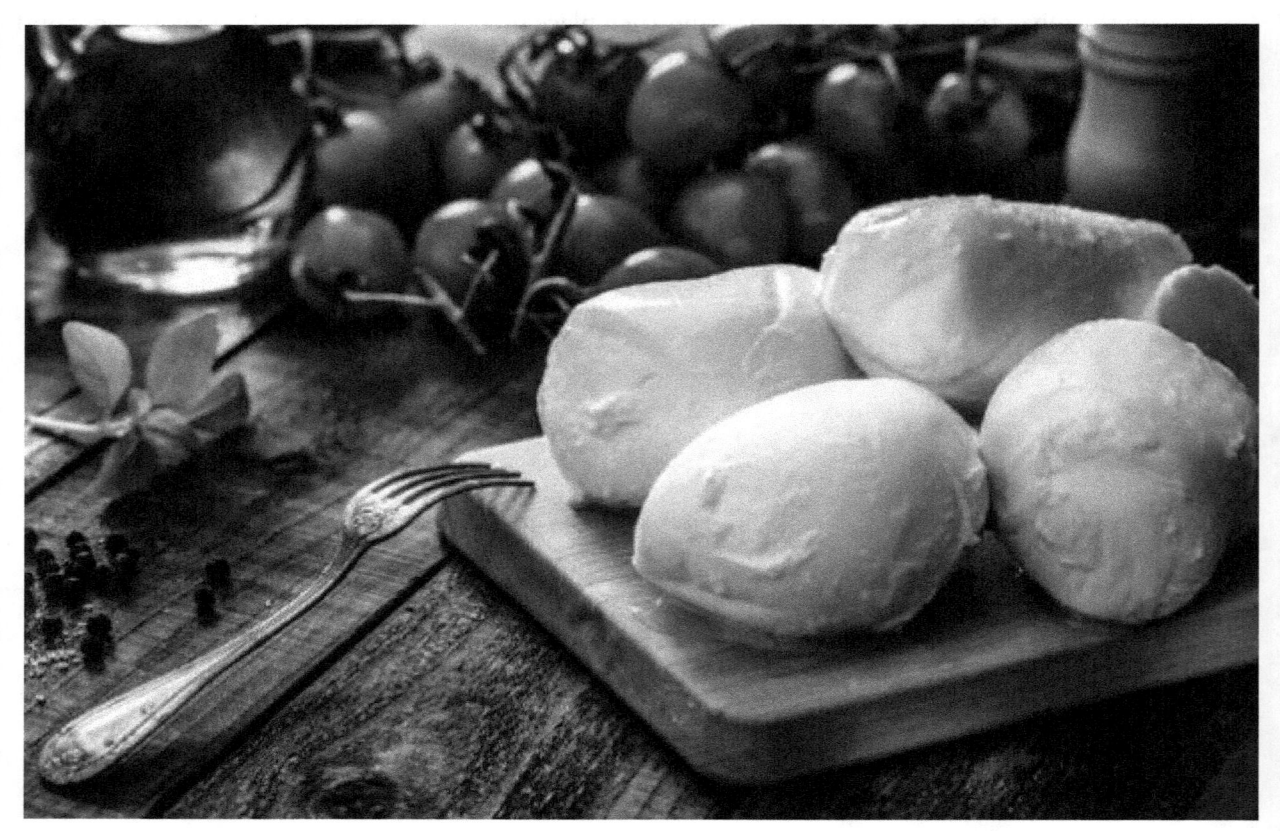

On the table you will see a fresh and fragrant addition to any Italian lunch or dinner that is traditional and as always, is super simple. See the gorgeous colors of the white juicy mozzarella bocconcini (bite-sized balls), tossed gently with the lovely green pesto and the vibrant red sun-blushed tomatoes.

The colors of Italy and a great beginner's dish to impress and improve.

<u>Total Prep Time</u>: 5 minutes

<u>Serving Size</u>: 6 servings

Ingredients	Measurements
Mozzarella bocconcini	2 cups
Olive oil	3 tbsp
Sun blushed tomatoes	½ cup
Grated parmesan	¼ cup
Fresh basil	2 cups
Pine nuts	1 tbsp
Garlic	1 clove
Salt and pepper	Small pinch

<u>Directions</u>:

1. With an immersion mixer (handheld mixer) or a mortar and pestle, combine the fresh basil, parmesan, garlic, and pine nuts. Mash it all up together into a paste that looks neither thick nor runny, but smooth and vibrant.
2. Now transfer the pesto into a bowl, drop in the mozzarella balls and drizzle over olive oil along with a pinch of salt and pepper, and there we go! It is ready to serve with some divine bread or on its own.

<u>Nifty Tips</u>:

● Make sure to take out the mozzarella from the fridge at least half an hour before preparation. The taste improves at room temperature. These are normally bought in a jar where they are brined and preserved (mozzarella di bufala), therefore it is important to strain them before use.

● Instead of sun-blushed tomatoes, you could also use sun-dried, but it would be better if you rehydrated them a little in warm water before including them into the meal as it might stand out as tough and excessively salty.

● I know pine nuts are ridiculously expensive these days, so you could alternatively use crushed pistachios, walnuts, or almonds, although the typical taste of pesto comes from the light and sweet flavor of pine nuts.

Focaccia With Walnuts

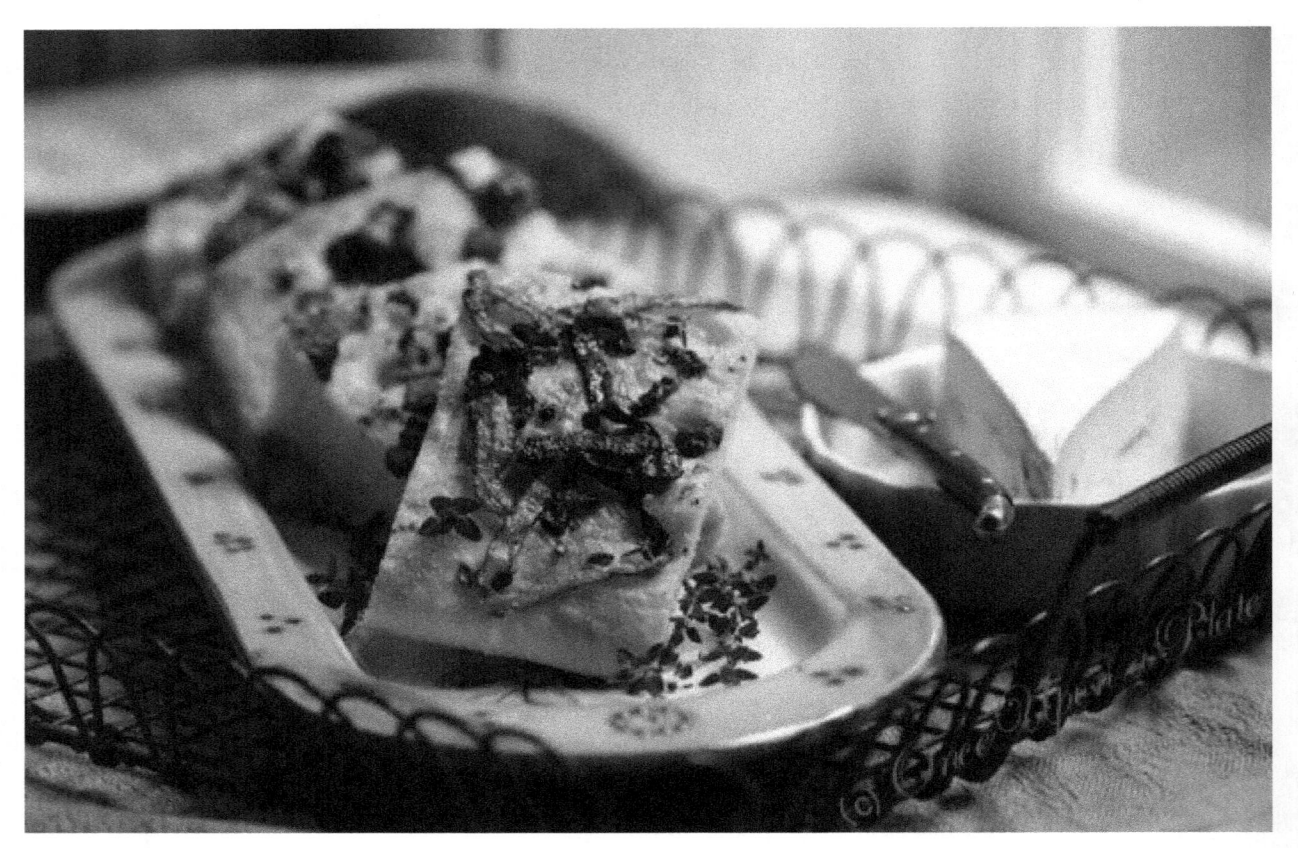

On the table, you will see focaccia that looks a little different from the rest. This focaccia is warm and inviting with gorgeous walnuts popping out of the crust just asking to be devoured. The nuttiness and subtle sweetness of the addition elevate the taste of this starter with incredible results.

Total: 3 hours and 45 minutes
Prep Time: 3 hours and 30 minutes (proofing included)
Baking Time: 15 minutes
Serving Size:

Ingredients	Measurements
Focaccia flour mix	As Chapter 5 recipe
Warm water	1 ⅓ + 1 tbsp
Olive oil	5 tbsp
Sugar	1 tsp
Walnut halves	1 cup

Directions:

1. In front of you, you should have the beginning flour mix consisting of AP flour, yeast, and salt. Add in

some sugar to resonate with the walnuts later when baking, careful to not let it touch the yeast in the bowl before mixing.
2. Roughly chop up the walnut halves into a size that is manageable. Not too big as to overpower the gluten network when baking. Combine well into the flour mix.
3. Pour in your warm water and olive oil and begin mixing it all together by hand into a rough ball.
4. On a floured surface, take the dough and begin kneading it for around 10 minutes to create a smooth network and elasticity.
5. From there you will follow the precise recipe as per my instructions in the previous chapter.

<u>Nifty Tips</u>:

- You can incorporate tomatoes, rosemary, or anything you like into a focaccia recipe.

Grissini

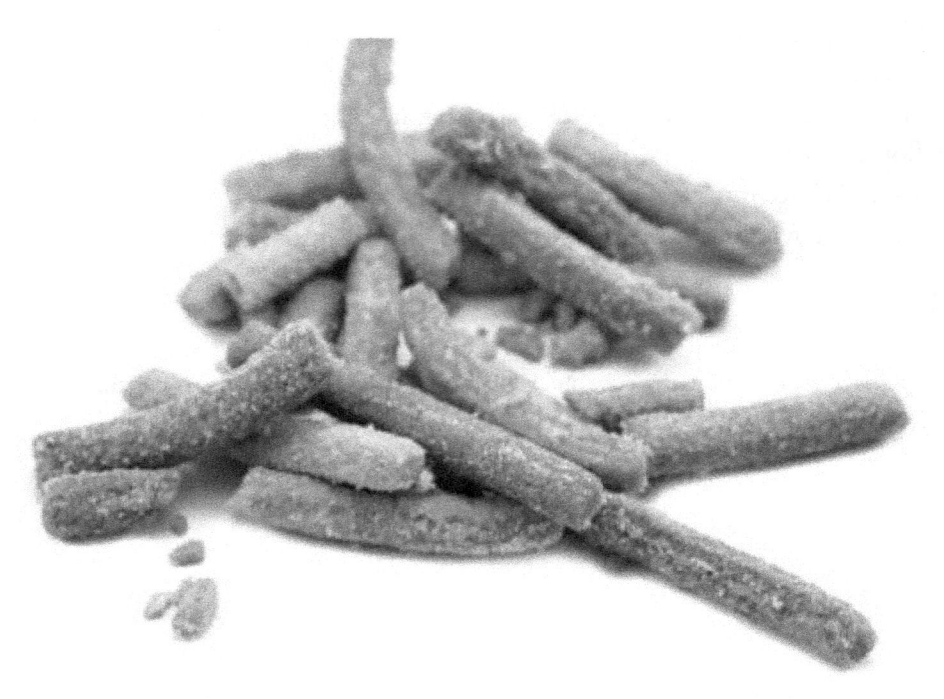

On the table you will see a weaved basket filled with long breadsticks, some covered in coarse salt, some with rosemary. They are perfect served as a starter with either cheese, olives, cured meat, or as is. This is one of my absolute favorites to keep around the house as a quick snack.

Total: 2 hours and 20 minutes
Prep Time: 1 hour and 50 minutes (proofing included)
Baking Time: 12 minutes
Serving Size: 20 breadsticks

Ingredients	Measurements
Bread flour	2 cups
Semolina flour	1 tbsp
Instant yeast	1 tsp
Warm water	¾ cups
Olive oil	2 tbsp
Sugar	1 tsp
Salt	1.5 tsp

Directions:

1. We will start by making the flour mix for the grissini. You will combine the flour, salt, and sugar into a bowl. With your hands, create a well in the center and insert the yeast, olive oil, and water.

2. Mix all of this together roughly into a doughy ball and place it on a floured surface. Knead the dough for around 10 minutes until you create that typical elastic and smooth consistency.
3. Place the dough into a bowl, sprinkle it lightly with flour, and cover it with plastic wrap for around 15 minutes to rest.
4. Remove the dough and place it on the floured surface to be shaped. The dough is pressed into a large rectangle. You will take each edge and fold it over itself in the middle like a letter.
5. The folded dough is then turned over, pinched at the edges to give it a more rectangular shape, and placed on a baking tray. Cover it once more to double in size for around 1 hour.
6. Preheat your oven at 450 °F (230 °C).
7. Once proofed sufficiently, uncover the baking tray and sprinkle some semolina on the dough and tray for easy cutting. Take the dough cutter and begin sectioning off ¼ inch pieces, widthwise, of the dough.
8. Shape each piece of dough gently into lengthy breadsticks, taking up as much space on the tray as possible without the pieces touching each other. Sprinkle semolina on the lengths.
9. Bake for around 15 minutes until you see the golden brown color rise. Once they have cooled down sufficiently, they are ready to be served.

<u>Nifty Tips</u>:

• It is best to use semolina or a harder bread flour to construct the grissini as it needs to hold a rough shape and keep a crispy texture. AP flour might make the texture too fine and crumbly.

• Of course, you can add things like chili flakes, red pepper flakes, garlic, rosemary, seeds, and coarse salt to the dough. Make two separate batches and test your taste buds.

Sautéed Prawns with Garlic And Chili

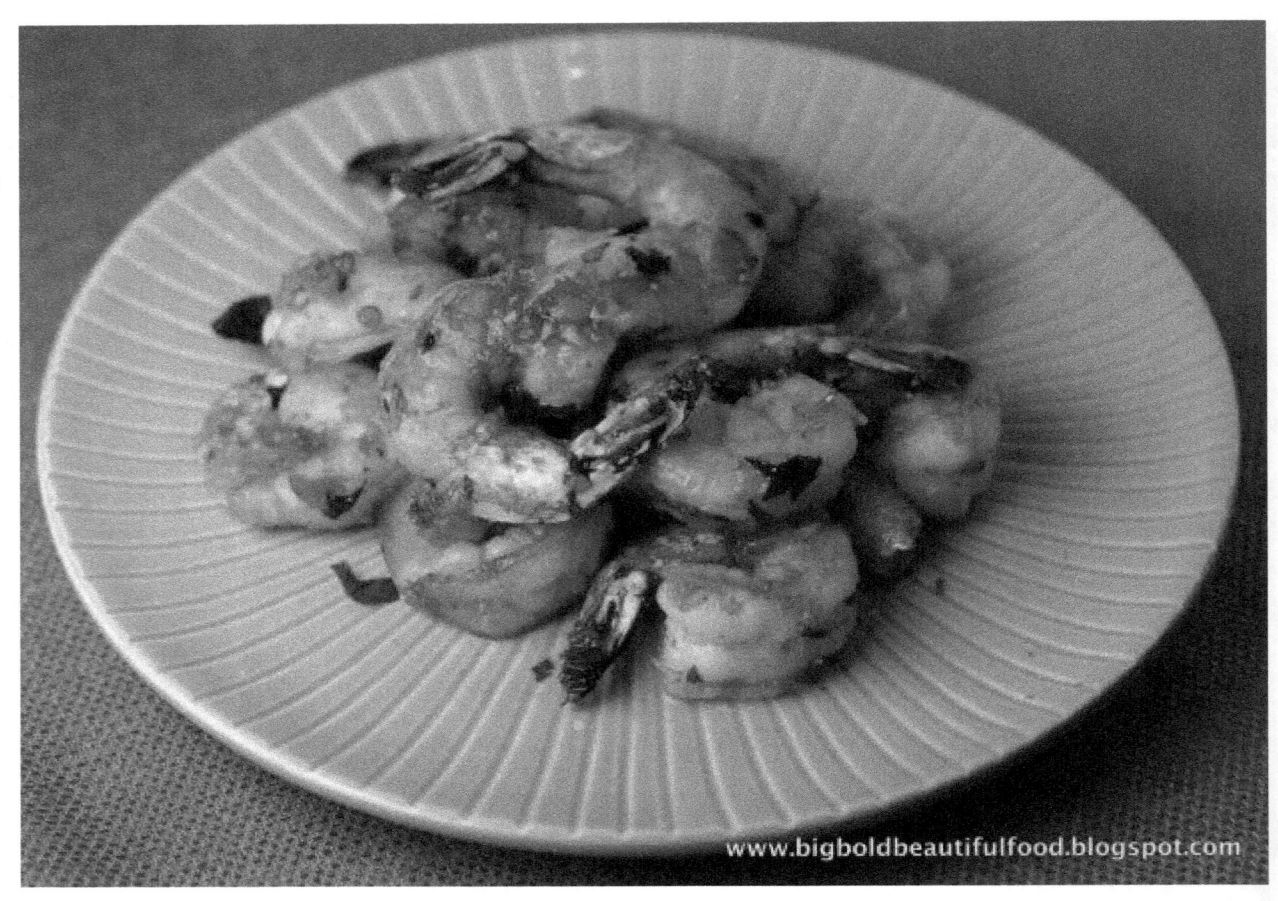

On the table you will see a vision of steaming pink prawns covered in fresh Italian colors like garlic, chili, and parsley. Served with some bread, this is one of the most decadent-looking starters that comes from good ingredients and easy work.

Total: 20 minutes
Prep Time: 10 minutes
Cooking Time: 10 minutes
Serving Size: 4 servings

Ingredients	Measurements
Raw and deveined king prawns	20
Garlic	2 large cloves
Fresh parsley	3 tbsp
Red chili peppers	2
Olive oil	3 tbsp
Lemon	1

Directions:

1. In a large frying pan, add olive oil and keep it at medium heat. Add 2 tbsp of chopped parsley and the finely sliced garlic. Deseed and slice up the chili, adding it to the mix as well. Fry gently until the garlic turns gold.
2. Add in the prawns, tossing continuously for around 3 minutes. Add some salt to taste.
3. Squeeze the lemon juice and sprinkle the lemon zest over the prawns while tossing for 1 more minute or so.
4. Remove from heat and plate, making sure to pour all the juice from the pan into the dish. Garnish with 1 tbsp of remaining parsley and serve hot.

Nifty Tips:

- If you do not have already deveined and peeled prawns, then it is important to clean them thoroughly before frying. They need to be fully defrosted and dried before putting into the pan or else they splatter and cook unevenly.

Genovese Mussels With Pesto and Olives

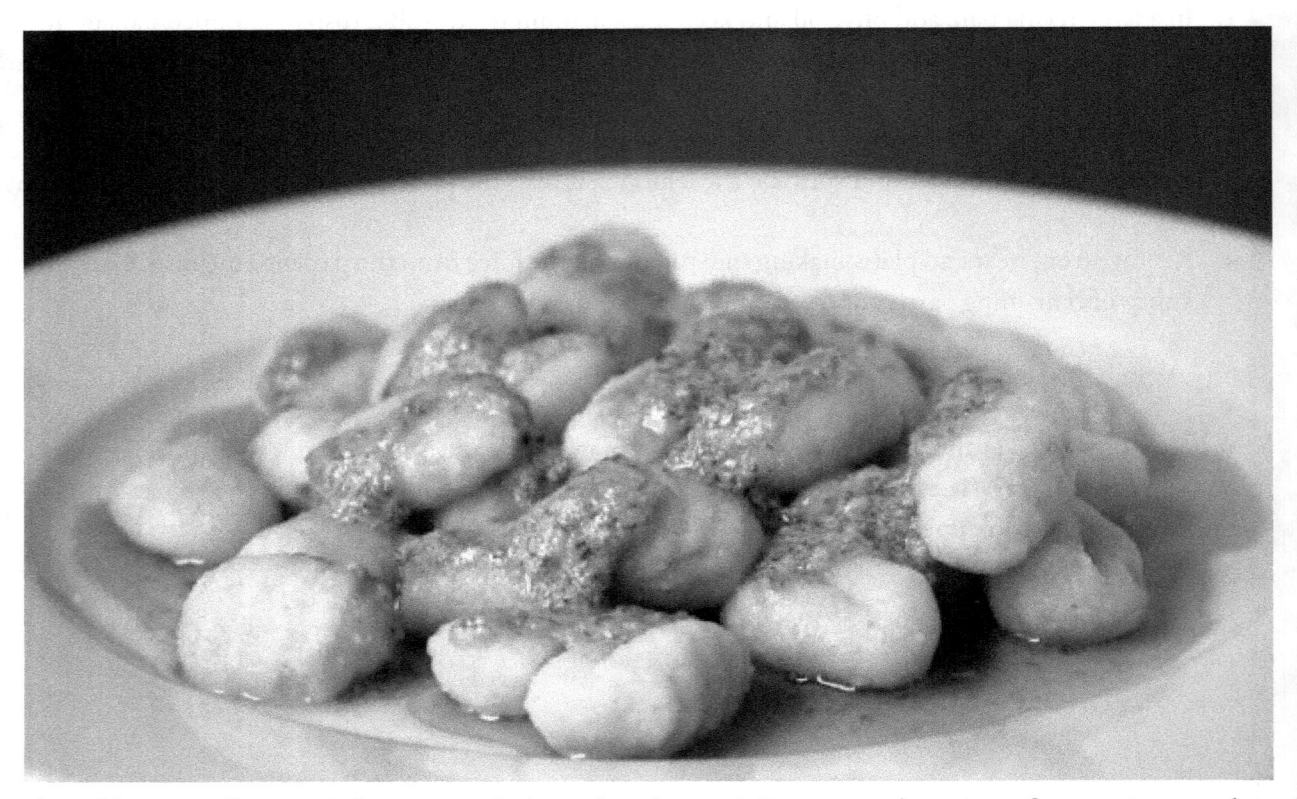

On the table you will see a skillet set on cloth, and within, a delicious combination of aromatic mussels and something else. What is that? Ah yes, the smell of pesto. And those are black olives scattered in the dish too. Well, there is no reason not to tuck in right away before it gets cold.

The combination is particular but worth a try, because if the Italians in Genoa do it, then it must be a hit.

<u>Total</u>: 23 minutes
<u>Prep Time</u>: 10 minutes
<u>Cooking Time</u>: 13 minutes
<u>Serving Size</u>: 4 servings

Ingredients	Measurements
Live mussels	2.6 lb
Cherry tomatoes	20
Garlic	4 cloves
Black olives	½ cup
Olive oil	4 tbsp
Fresh basil	10 leaves
Pesto	3 tbsp
White wine	½ cup
Salt and pepper	Pinch

<u>Directions</u>:

1. The importance of cleaning mussels properly should not be overlooked. Begin by placing them under cold running water and scrubbing them with a new scrubbing brush. Remove all debris, making sure the hairs and sand are gone, and remove the fluffy beards that sprout from the stem.
2. Once cleaned and set aside to dry, you can begin heating a large pan at medium heat with olive oil. Add the sliced garlic and drained olives and when they are sizzling, throw in the mussels. This is tossed and stirred continuously for around 2 minutes.
3. Next you will increase the heat to high and add in the white wine. Stir every so often for another 3 minutes to allow the wine to reduce.
4. Close the lid and let it simmer for another 3 minutes, shaking the pan occasionally to open the shells. Discard the mussels that refuse to open.
5. When all the shells are open, you can add in your cherry tomatoes, fresh basil, pesto, and salt and pepper. Stir on and off for a further 5 minutes to incorporate the flavors. Then it is ready to serve from the pan into bowls. Yum!

<u>Nifty Tips</u>:

- If you buy store-bought mussels, frozen or fresh, you will have an easier time cleaning them due to less dirt present in the tanks.

- Make sure to knock on the shells while washing them to check if they are all alive. If they do not move and shift in their shell, then the mussel needs to be discarded. The same goes for broken shells.

- I always recommend using unpitted olives for extra flavor and meatiness.

- You could easily make your own pesto, but for the convenience of the recipe, I am using a purchased jar.

Fried Baby Artichokes

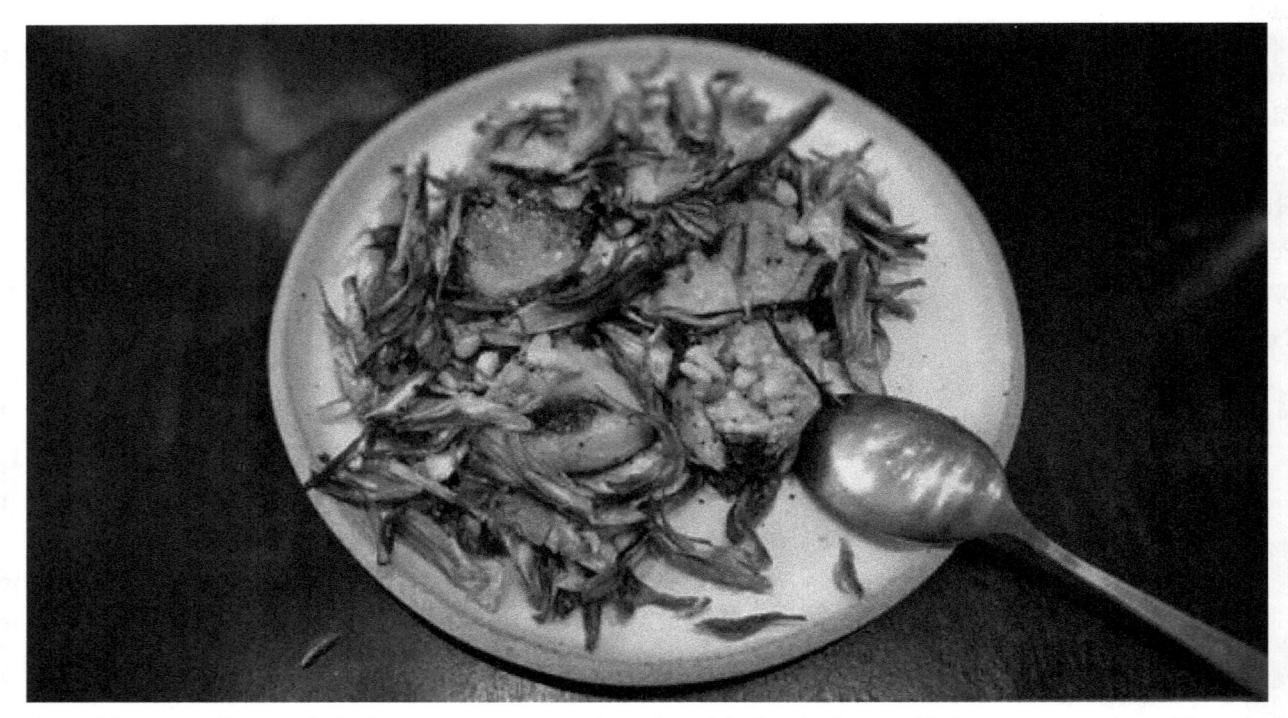

On the table you will see a dish that contains something lavishly fried; the smell alone is rewarding. These baby artichokes are deep-fried to perfection and topped with parmesan cheese and parsley to elevate the flavor.

This is a typical and beloved Roman appetizer that brings you closer to Italy with each bite.

Total: 23 minutes

Prep Time: 15 minutes

Cooking Time: 8 minutes

Serving Size: 10 servings

Ingredients	Measurements
Baby artichokes	20 (80 oz)
Parmesan	¼ cup
Fresh parsley	¼ cup
Olive oil	½ cup
Salt and pepper	Pinch

Directions:

1. Start by preparing the artichokes for frying. Wash and chop off any stems. Peel away outer leaves until you reach the tender inner leaves, and chop off the tip of the artichoke. This leaves you with a trimmed and tender baby artichoke that you will then quarter lengthwise.
2. In a large pan, heat the olive oil at a high temperature. Place the artichokes into the oil in batches of 5

until they are crispy and light, which is around 2 minutes per batch.
3. Sprinkle some salt and pepper onto the batch as they drain on paper towels before serving with grated parmesan and finely chopped parsley.

Classic Bruschetta With Tomato and Basil

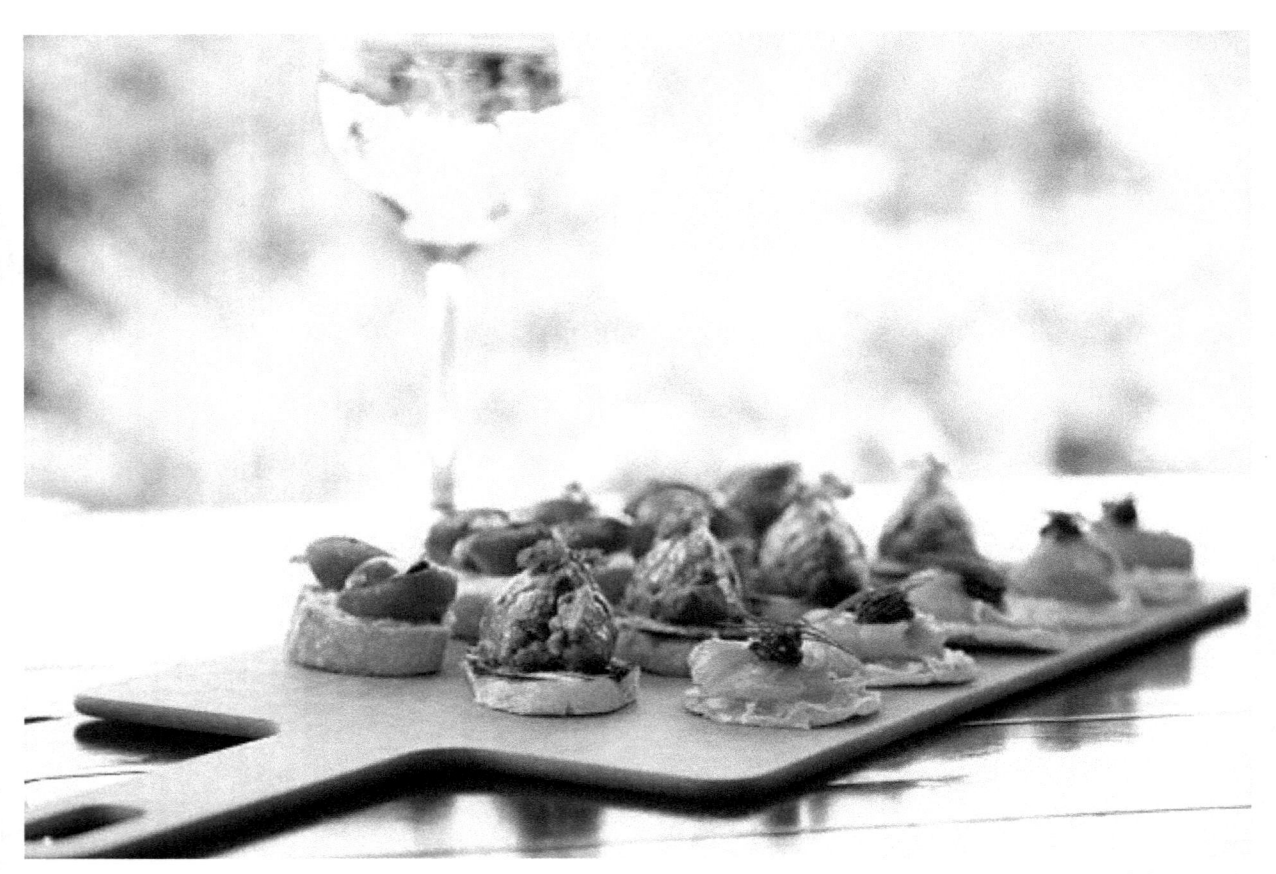

On the table you will see what can only be described as the original and undisputed champion of the quick Italian snack: the humble bruschetta. The tomato and basil work together wonderfully and elevate the crispy and airy Italian baguette to new heights.

This is the simplest of combinations and the best starter or snack to not overwhelm but to fulfill.

Total: 40 minutes

Prep Time: 30 minutes

Cooking Time: 10 minutes

Serving Size: 15 servings

Ingredients	Measurements
Italian or French baguette	1 large
Roma tomatoes	10 (2 lb)
White onion	¼ cup
Basil	¼ cup
Garlic	2 cloves
Balsamic vinegar	2 tsp
Olive oil	1 tbsp
Salt and pepper	Pinch

<u>Directions</u>:

1. Begin by grabbing your cleaned tomatoes, de-seeding them, and dicing them up into a medium texture. Add them to a bowl with the minced onion, 1 minced garlic clove, balsamic vinegar, and thinly sliced basil. Mix well with 1 tbsp of olive oil, salt, and pepper.
2. Preheat your oven to 450 °F (232 °C).
3. Grab your bread knife and slice up the baguette into ½ inch to ¾ inch thick slices. Brush over olive oil and sprinkle salt on each side of the slice. Place them on your lined baking tray and bake for approximately 10 minutes, turning over halfway through.
4. When out of the oven, take the other garlic clove, cut it in half, and rub it into one side of the bruschetta to infuse aroma and flavor.
5. Spoon out the tomato and basil sauce onto the crispy and warm bruschetta and it is ready to serve.

<u>Nifty Tips</u>:

- You could literally add anything under the sun on top of a crispy bruschetta, so get creative and use anchovies, olives, various other cured meats, cheeses, and spreads.

Fried Sage Leaves With Anchovies

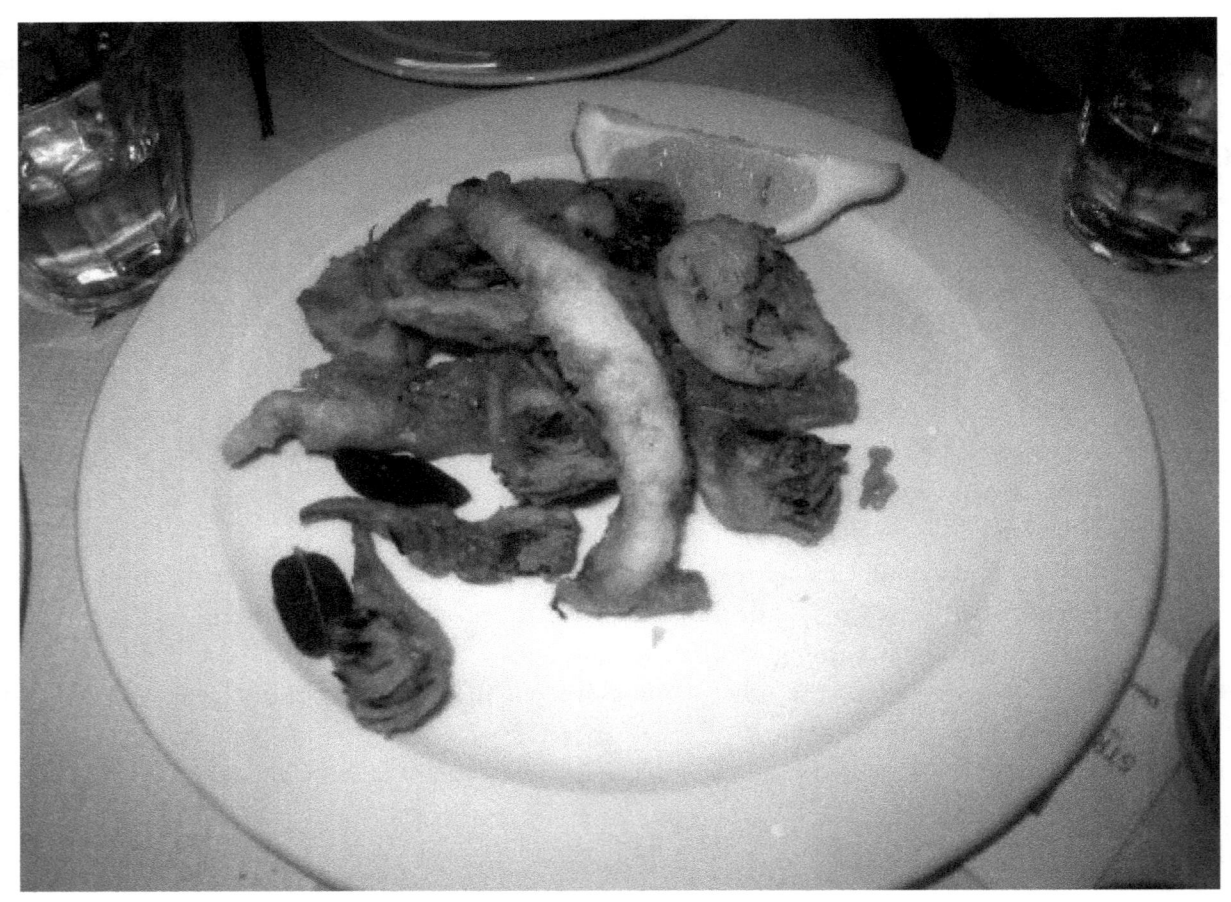

On the table you will see a plate filled with something green and fried. It looks absolutely mouth-watering and you can smell the rich and salty aroma of anchovy along with the subtle sweet smell of fried sage. Together it is a sight that no one can resist.

This combo is a punch of flavor and a great summer snack served with some sparkling wine.

<u>Total</u>: 18 minutes

<u>Prep Time</u>: 10 minutes

<u>Cooking Time</u>: 8 minutes

<u>Serving Size</u>: 4 servings

Ingredients	Measurements
Anchovy filets	12
Sage leaves	24
AP flour	4 tbsp
Sparkling water	⅓ cup + 1 tbsp
Sunflower oil	Frying
Lemon	1

Directions:

1. We begin by making sure the anchovies are rinsed enough of all their salt and oil. Drain and dry them down thoroughly to prevent splattering.
2. Handle your anchovies depending on the size of your sage leaves, cutting them in half if need be. They need to be able to fit snugly between 2 leaves, sandwiched in and pinched closed.
3. In a hot deep frying pan, pour in your oil and let heat up.
4. Start your batter by whisking in a medium bowl the flour and sparkling water until a smooth and runny texture is achieved.
5. Quickly and efficiently dip your anchovy and sage parcels in the batter, covering all sides, and then put them into the hot and bubbling oil. Fry batches until they are floating and golden on each side.
6. Place fried parcels onto a paper towel to drain and serve with a pinch of salt and quartered lemon wedges to bring acidity to the dish.

Nifty Tips:

- Cleaning the anchovies of all the excess salt is important. The punch of saltiness can be overwhelming when deep-fried.

- The batter should be of a consistency that is runny but still clings to the sage leaves before frying.

- You could very well use normal water to make the batter, but the aeration from sparkling water allows it to fluff up and crisp better.

Chapter 7: Ricotta

I would like to focus a little on the soft and smooth cheese that can be so easy to make and so versatile. Yup, that would be ricotta cheese!

We have already taken a look at the basic recipe in Chapter 5, and I would like to show you here how you can zhuzh things up a tad and incorporate some kickass flavors to the subtle cheese.

Whether it be lavishly spread over some crispy bread or as the main ingredient for specialty dishes, this cheese will show you exactly what it's worth. The more you make it, the better you will become at deciding where to use it. Young and mature ricotta each have their own value and I would like to bring to your repertoire five gorgeous recipes to try at home now!

Whipped Ricotta Dip With Cherry Tomatoes

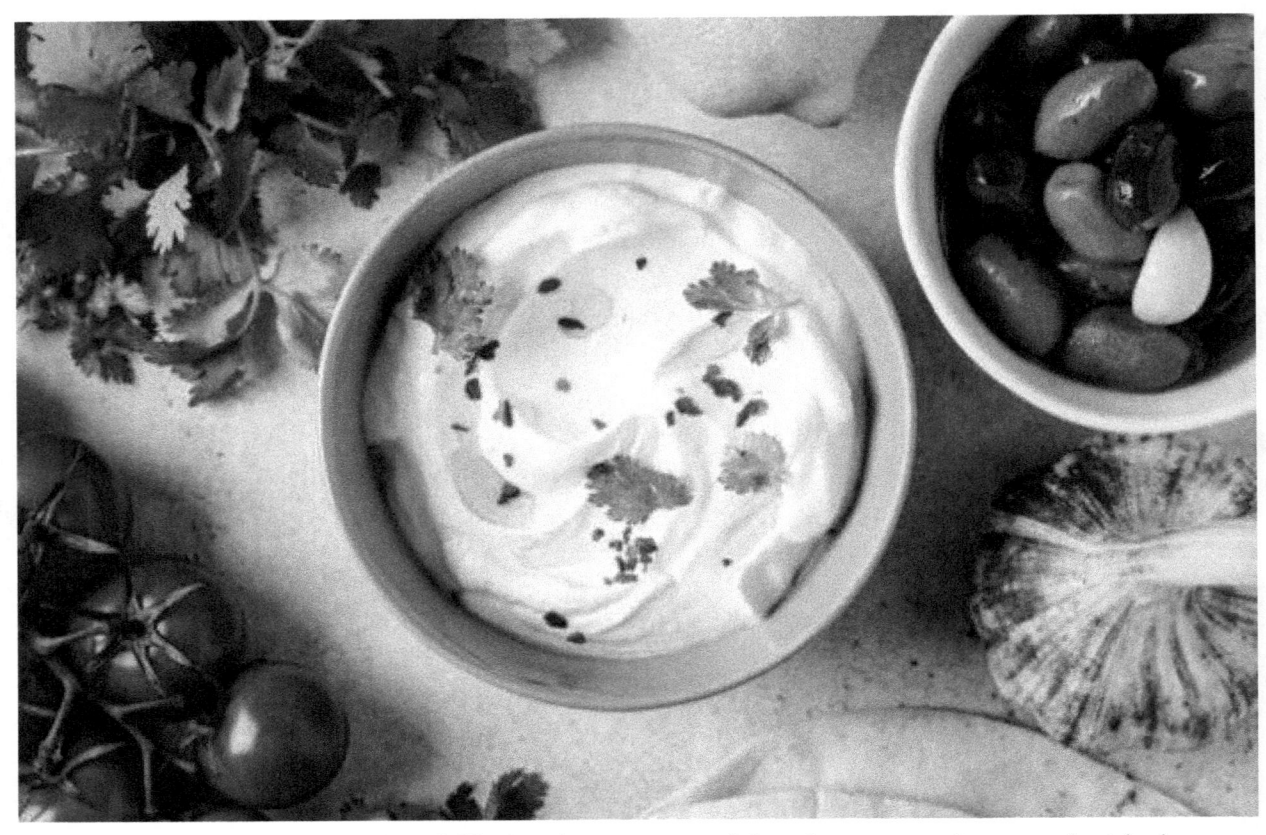

On the table you will see a serving bowl filled with a creamy and decadent ricotta dip topped with char-roasted and deliciously juicy cherry tomatoes.

This is a delightful snack when served with raw vegetable sticks or crunchy bread slices. Dip and go, so that you have one hand free for a glass of wine.

Total: 30 minutes
Prep Time: 5 minutes
Cooking Time: 20 minutes
Serving Size: 8 servings

Ingredients	Measurements
Full fat ricotta	1 cup
Cherry tomatoes	1.5 cups
Parmesan cheese	2 tbsp
Thyme	1 tbsp
Olive oil	1 tbsp
Lemon	1
Salt and pepper	Pinch

Special Equipment:

- Food processor

Directions:

1. Begin by preheating your oven to 350 °F (180°C).
2. On a baking tray, lay your halved cherry tomatoes, drizzle ½ tbsp of olive oil, and sprinkle the thyme, salt, and pepper for taste. Pop into the oven for between 15 and 20 minutes then set aside to cool.
3. In your food processor blitz up the ricotta, lemon zest, grated parmesan cheese, and some salt and pepper until you get a soft and creamy texture.
4. When serving, place the dip into a bowl and make a small well in the center. Spoon in the roasted tomatoes and a drizzle of olive oil. Delish!

Nifty Tips:

- This will usually last around 2 to 3 days in the fridge if covered.

Baked Ricotta With Thyme and Parmesan

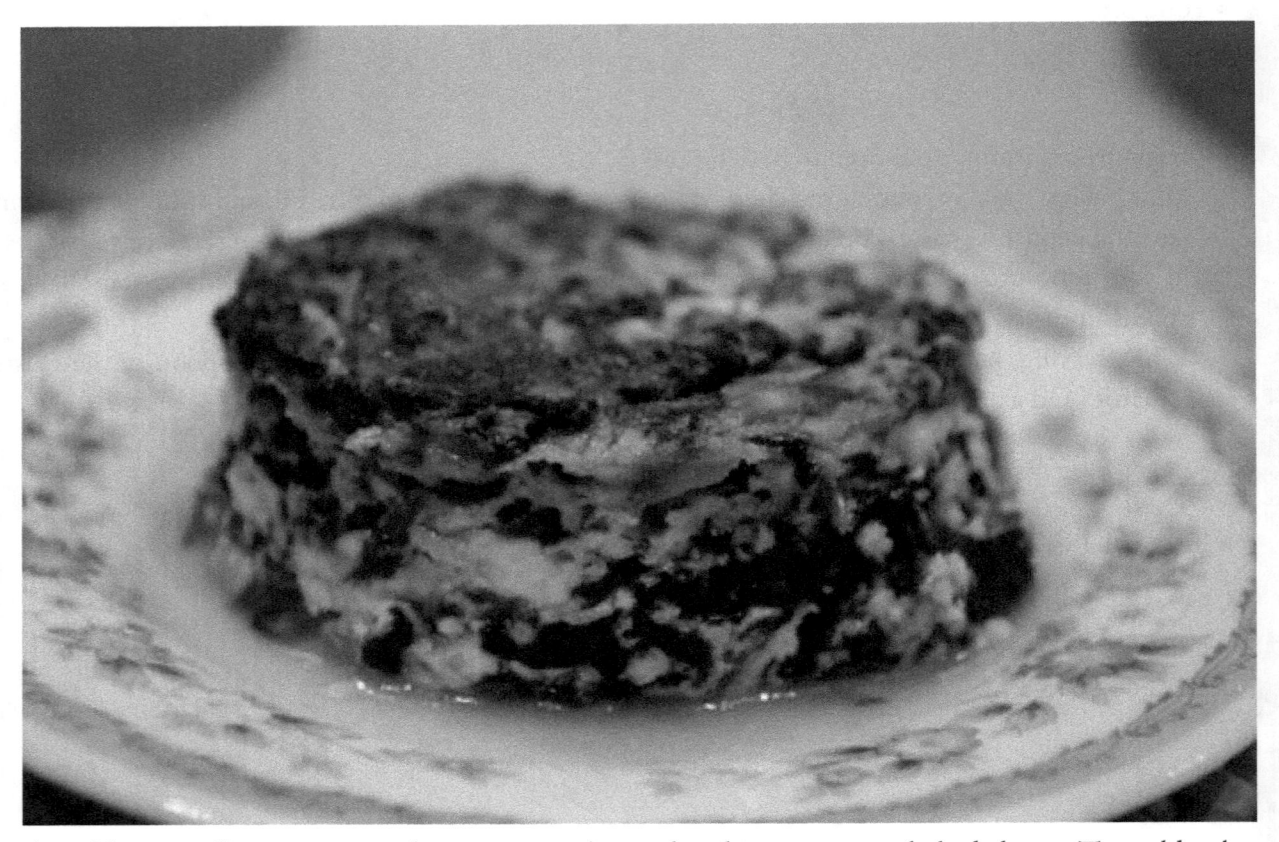

On the table you will see a warm and inviting ramekin and within it a creamy baked cheese. The golden-brown crust hides a soft and aromatic center infused with thyme and parmesan.

With a spoon, spread on bread or serve alongside baked vegetables and sliced meats.

<u>Total</u>: 35 minutes

<u>Prep Time</u>: 5 minutes

<u>Cooking Time</u>: 30 minutes

<u>Serving Size</u>: 4 servings

Ingredients	Measurements
Full fat ricotta	2 cups
Eggs	2
Parmesan	1 cup
Fresh thyme	1 tbsp
Nutmeg	Pinch
Butter	Greasing

<u>Special Equipment</u>:

- Baking ramekins

Directions:

1. Let's start by preheating the oven at 400 °F (200 °C).
2. Grease your ramekins with butter and set them aside.
3. Squeeze out as much excess moisture from the ricotta as possible before you place it in a mixing bowl or food processor and give it a good whisk till smooth.
4. Add in the eggs and combine further.
5. Add the chopped thyme, the grated parmesan, and a sprinkle of nutmeg and salt and pepper. Mix well.
6. Into the buttered ramekins, spoon out ¾ of the dish with your mix and use the back of your spoon to even out the surface. Bake for around 35 minutes till puffed up and golden. Serve and delight.

Nifty Tips:

- Strain the ricotta using either a strainer and a spoon or pressure from a cheesecloth.

- The beauty of ricotta is that you can enjoy it straight from the oven or the next day when it's cold. Both are divine!

- This dish could easily be prepared a day earlier and then just popped into the oven the next.

Spinach and Ricotta Egg Pie

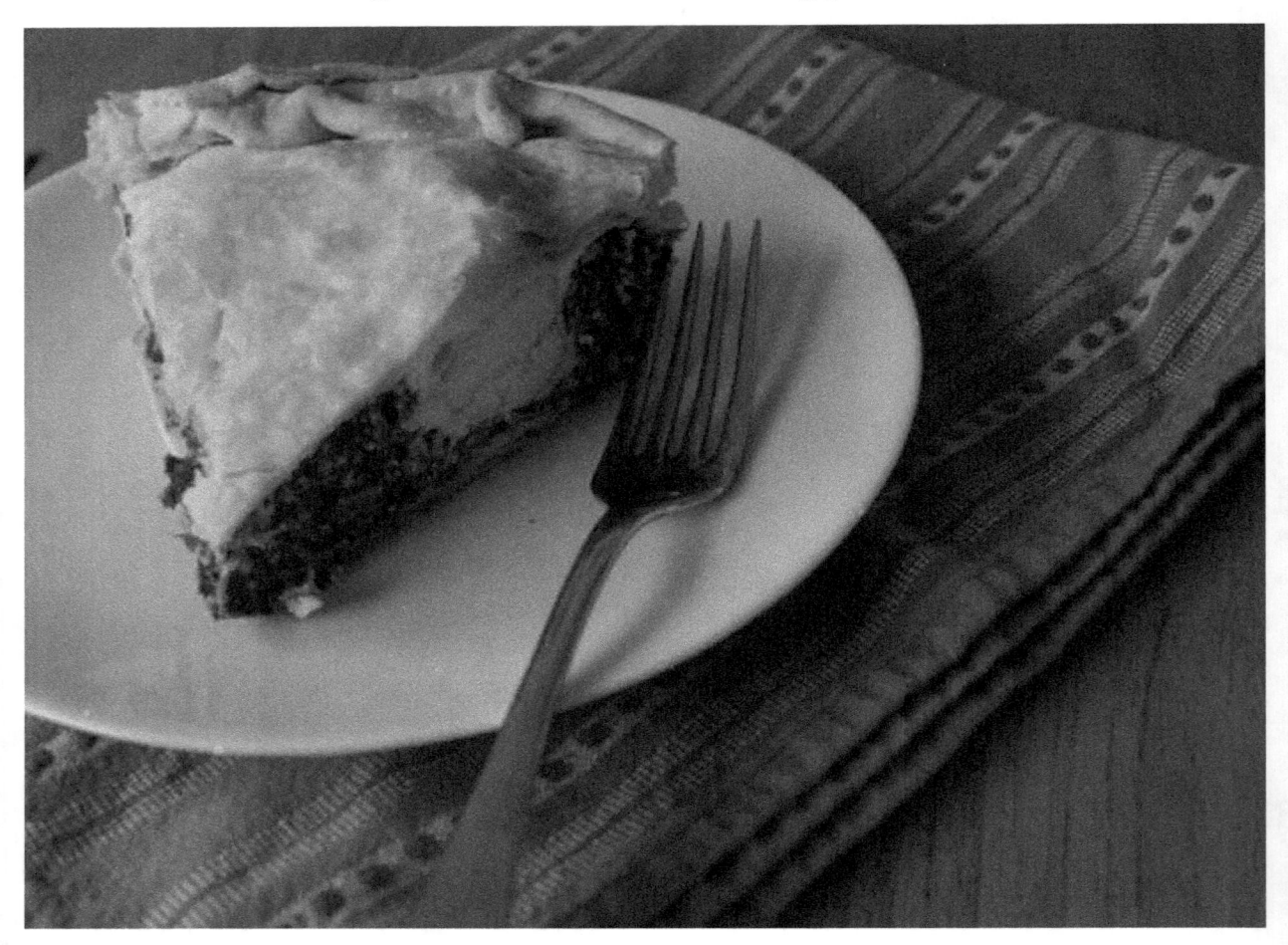

On the table you will see a typical dish eaten on Easter in Italy; *la torta pasqualina*. This pie is super crusty and when you cut through the puff pastry you are greeted by the ricotta and spinach fillings with whole eggs nestled within. It is so pretty and creative it's a must on special occasions.

<u>Total</u>: 1 hour 20 minutes
<u>Prep Time</u>: 20 minutes
<u>Cooking Time</u>: 1 hour
<u>Serving Size</u>: 12 servings

Ingredients	Measurements
Puff pastry	1.5 lb
Full-fat ricotta	2 cups
Baby spinach	2 cups
Eggs	5
Brown onion	1
Garlic	2 cloves
Pecorino	1 cup
Olive oil	2 tbsp
Butter	Greasing
Nutmeg	Pinch
Salt and pepper	Pinch

Directions:

1. Take the puff pastry out of the fridge, then grease the interior of a large 9-inch pie dish with butter.
2. In a large pan, heat ½ tbsp of olive oil and sauté your finely chopped onion until glassy. Then, add in your chopped garlic until golden and finally your spinach leaves.
3. Let this wilt for around 5 minutes then take the spinach mix off the heat and place somewhere to cool down.
4. When it has sufficiently cooled, you can begin finely chopping the spinach then adding it to a large mixing bowl. Spoon in the ricotta and sprinkle in the nutmeg and salt and pepper. Adequately combine till firm and creamy and set aside.
5. Preheat your oven to 350 °F (180 °C). Your puff pastry should be at room temperature, making it easier to mold in the pie dish.
6. Cover the interior of the pie dish with the pastry, making sure to push it into the corners without breaking it. Cut the edges.
7. Dollop out the spinach and cheese mixture evenly into the dish. With the back of a spoon, create four equally spaced indentations in the spinach mix. Crack four of your eggs into those predisposed spaces.
8. Now cover the entire mix with another layer of puff pastry and fold in the edges to seal the pie.
9. Whisk your remaining egg into an egg wash to brush over the surface of the pie and poke a small hole in the crust center for escaping steam while baking.
10. Bake for 50 minutes carefully watching as the crust darkens to a golden hue. Let it cool completely before you serve.

Nifty Tips:

- Do not overcook your spinach or whichever kind of green you choose, as you still want some moisture in the filling. Just as it begins to wilt, remove from the heat.

- If the egg bed is too shallow, the egg cracked within will spill over and not give the desired look after baking.

Crostini With Ricotta and Peas

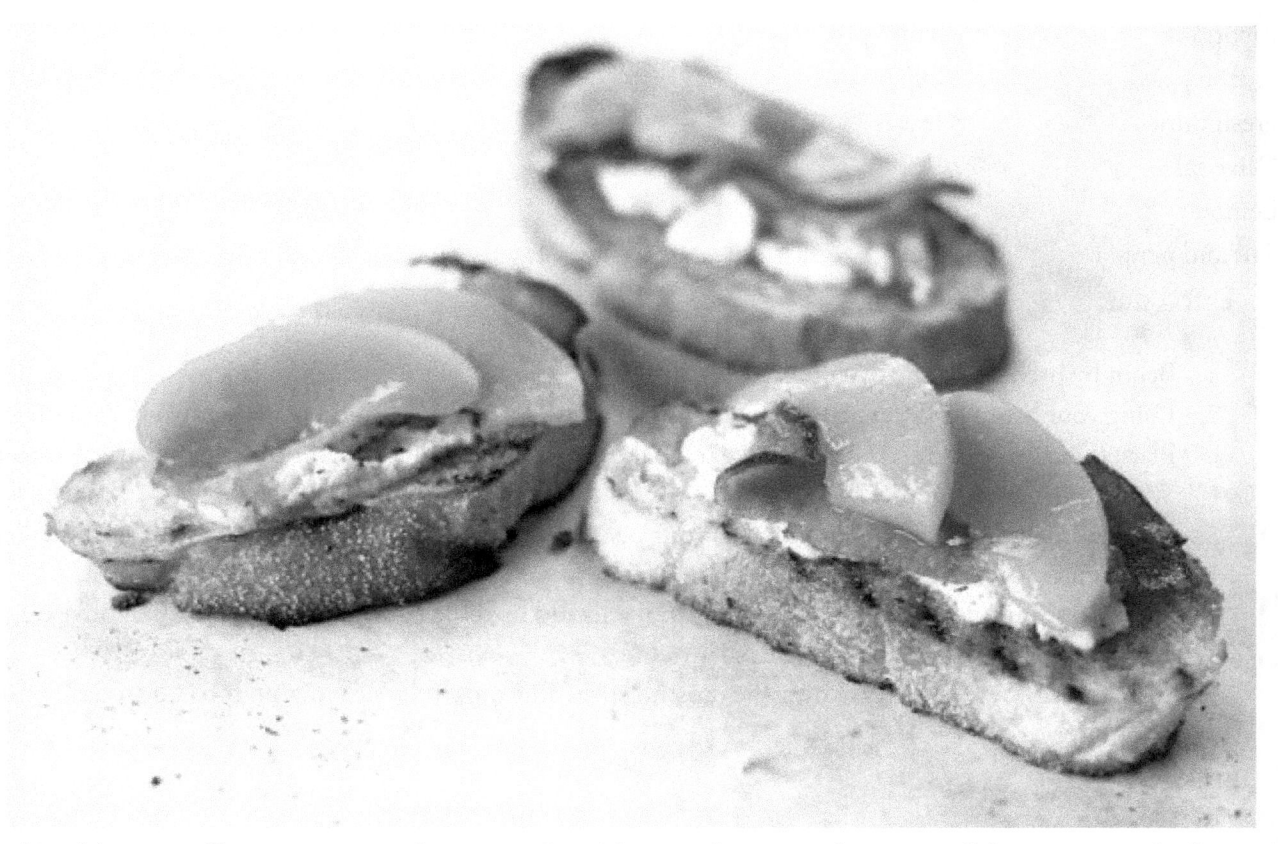

On the table you will see your typical crostini charred to perfection and on top of that is a spread of ricotta cheese and vibrant green peas. How interesting! As you bite in, you will savor the soft cheese with pops of sweetness from the peas and acidity from the lemon zest. Divine.

What a lovely summer snack perfect for a quick afternoon get-together.

Total: 27 minutes

Prep Time: 15 minutes

Cooking Time: 12 minutes

Serving Size: 12 servings

Ingredients	Measurements
Italian or French baguette	1 large loaf
Ricotta	½ cup
Frozen peas	1 cup
Fresh mint	8 leaves
Olive oil	2 tbsp
Lemon	1/2
Salt and pepper	Pinch

<u>Directions:</u>

1. Begin by preheating the oven to 340 °F (170 °C).
2. Using your bread knife, cut the baguette into ½ inch slices, and brush the slices with ½ tbsp of olive oil. Place them on your lined baking sheet and bake for around 10 minutes, turning them halfway through. When crispy, remove and let cool.
3. Bring a small pot to a boil and blanch your peas for 2 minutes until tender. Wash them immediately under cold water and place them in a bowl.
4. Shred your mint leaves, zest your lemon rind, and add it to the peas, along with 1 tbsp of olive oil, salt, and pepper. Gently mix to infuse flavors well.
5. Now spread the fresh ricotta over the crostini slices and spoon the pea mix on top. Add a dash of olive oil and serve.

Ricotta Gnocchi

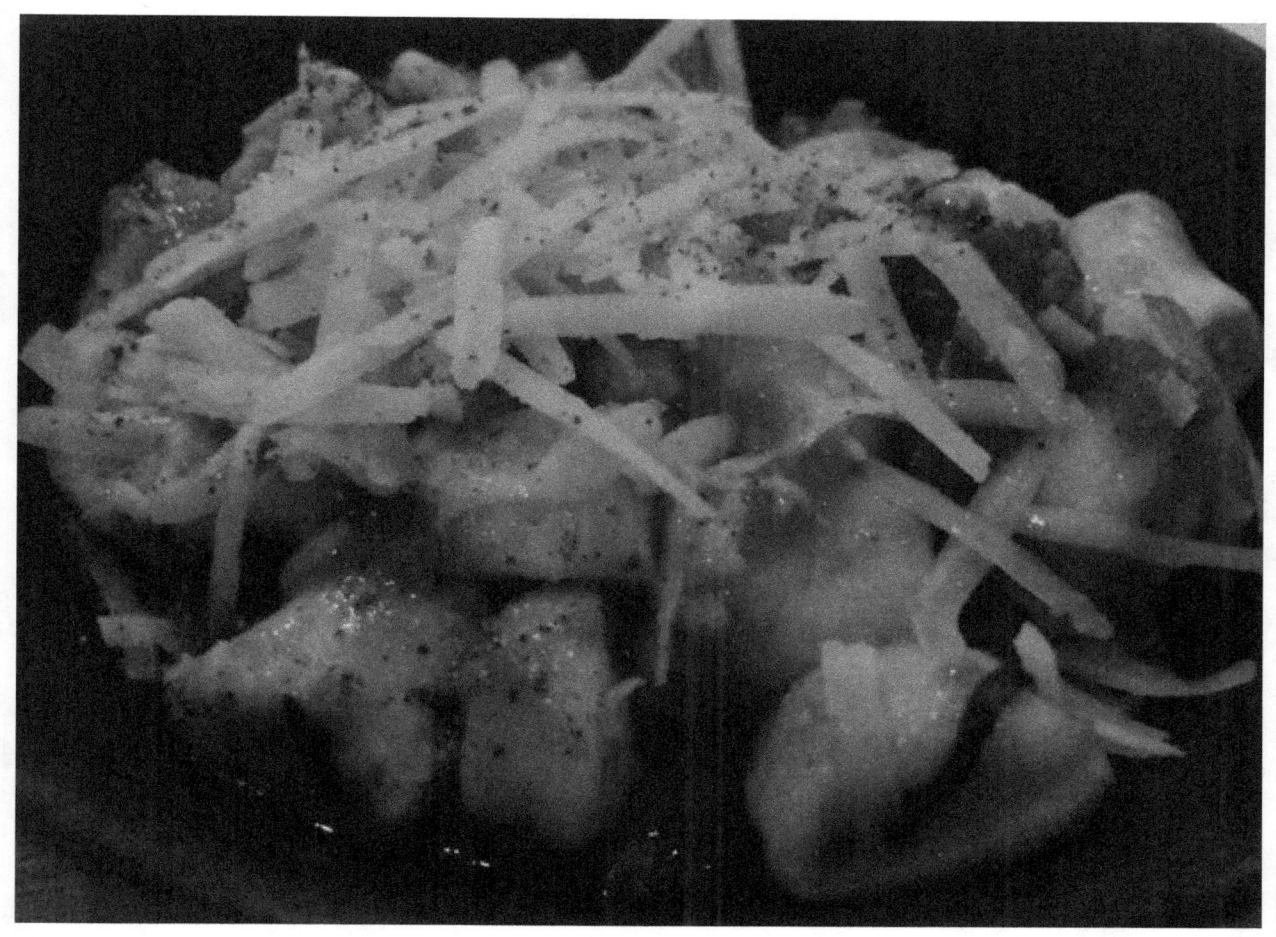

On the table you will see a plate jumping with enthusiasm: yellow gnocchi nestled into a tomato and cheese sauce. Fresh, yet hearty. This is a wonderful lunchtime meal that gets you fed and happy in no time.

<u>Total</u>: 38 minutes

<u>Prep Time</u>: 30 minutes

<u>Cooking Time</u>: 8 minutes

<u>Serving Size</u>: 4 servings

Ingredients	Measurements
Full-fat ricotta	1 ½ cups (8 oz)
AP flour	1 cup
Eggs	2
Marinara sauce	2 cups
Parmesan	½ cup
Olive oil	½ tbsp
Fresh basil	Handful
Salt and pepper	Pinch

Special Equipment:

- Kitchen scale
- Bench scraper

Directions:

1. We should begin by ensuring the ricotta cheese is sufficiently drained. We will need to make sure the weight is correct by placing the dried ricotta on a kitchen scale. On a scale set to zero, place within a bowl the dried ricotta, ensuring you reach an 8 oz weight.
2. Within that bowl, add in your grated parmesan and half of your flour.
3. Take 1 egg and separate it, discarding the egg white. Add that egg yolk to the bowl along with the other whole egg. Add a touch of salt and pepper and begin mixing with preferably a rubber spatula. The mixture should be of a sticky texture, but not necessarily loose. Add more flour if the mixture is too wet and sticky.
4. Now begin shaping the dough on a lightly floured surface. Take your whole mixture and roughly shape it into a rectangle. Using your bench scraper, divide the dough into 4 segments.
5. Each segment should be gently rolled into a log of around 12 inches in length and about ¾ inch in width. Cut each log into around 10 equal portions.
6. In a large pot, bring salt water to a boil. Cook the gnocchi until they begin to float, then after 30 seconds, remove them and drain. Keep ½ cup of pasta water.
7. In another pan, heat up your marinara sauce, and add in the drained gnocchi. Add in your pasta water to emulsify the lot.
8. Serve and garnish with more grated cheese and chopped fresh basil.

Nifty Tips:

- You could use any herb you think is best. Adding parsley or fresh chives works well too.

- Using thick paper towels to absorb the moisture of the ricotta is a good idea. The ricotta needs to be very well-drained and dried.

- Gnocchi can be frozen directly in flour-dusted zip lock bags for around 2 months.

- Be careful not to oversaturate the dough with flour as that would not bring about the best results when cooking. Gnocchi should be sticky but easy to handle. Dust off if necessary.

Chapter 8: Zuppe [Soups]

If there is one thing that brings me joy, it's a quality soup made with love and TLC. Whether served warm or cold, I can appreciate the different flavors coming together, and plus it's super healthy for you!

Just as we keep good friends around us to better our lives, so we should also keep good ingredients around us to better our food. The simplest of methods cannot stop a perfectly ripe and juicy Roma tomato from bringing life to a soup. Anything can be blitzed together and called a soup, but if your foundation is solid, it can be called a great soup!

Depending on the region in which it originates, it can be seen as a chunky meaty soup or a smooth and creamy soup. We will have a look at a little bit of it all.

Zuppa Toscana

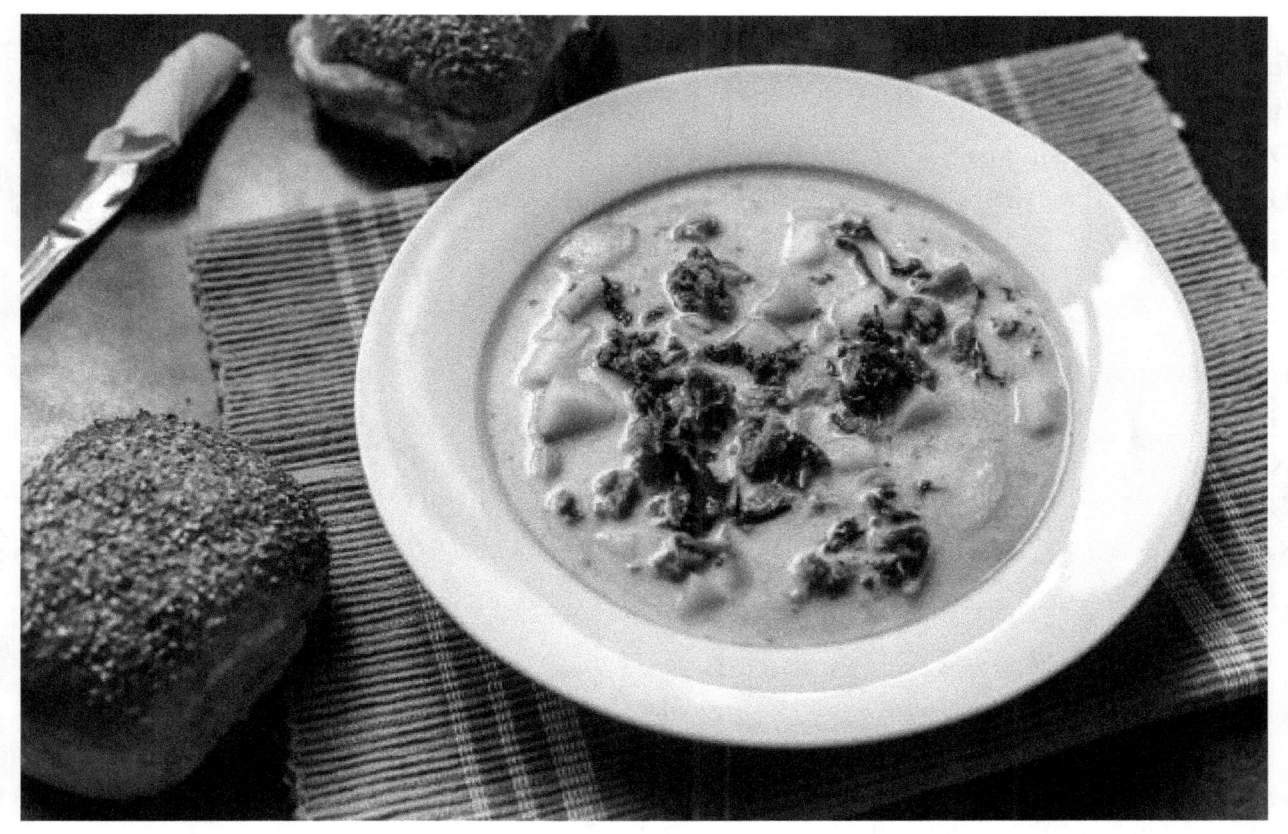

On the table you will see a bowl of warm inviting soup. The creamy base will smell divine, and as you investigate further you will find a plentiful of lovely ingredients swimming happily within: the texture of the potatoes, the richness of the sausage and cream, then the fresh tang of kale and beans.

This is warm and soulful, absolutely perfect for cold winter nights.

<u>Total</u>: 1 hour 30 minutes

<u>Prep Time</u>: 30 minutes (excludes soaking time)

<u>Cooking Time</u>: 1 hour

<u>Serving Size</u>: 16 servings

Ingredients	Measurements
Fresh kale	1 head
Idaho potatoes	3 medium
Italian sausage	2 lb
Bacon	8 slices
Dried cannellini beans	1 bag
Heavy cream	1 ½ cups
Yellow onion	1
Carrots	2
Celery	3 sticks
Parmesan rinds	3
Garlic	5 cloves
AP flour	¼ cup
Chicken stock	96 oz
Salt and pepper	Pinch

Directions:

1. You want to first make sure you soak your beans overnight in water so they soften adequately.
2. Preheat your oven to 400 °F (205 °C) and place the bacon slices on a lined baking tray.
3. In a large pan at medium heat, add some olive oil and cook your sausage till well done.
4. In that time, the bacon should be cooking in the oven for 15 to 20 minutes until crispy. Remove sausage from pan and set aside and remove bacon from oven to cool as well.
5. In that same pan, add your diced onion, carrots, celery sticks, and finely minced garlic to cook in the sausage fat and sweat. 7 minutes at medium to low heat should do the trick.
6. Shake your flour into the pan and combine slowly with the vegetables. Once evenly mixed, add in your sausage, parmesan rinds, drained beans, and chicken stock to simmer at low heat for 30 minutes.
7. Wash and slice the potatoes around ⅓ inch thick then quarter them and drop them into the pan. Let it all cook together for a further 10 minutes.
8. Finally, you will gently mix in the whipped cream, chopped crispy bacon, and salt and pepper. Serve with a couple of leaves of fresh kale so it wilts while being eaten. Perfect!

Nifty Tips:

- You can easily swap your chicken stock for beef stock.

- When working with beans in a meal, it is always best to soak them overnight in warm water. This allows the outer shell to soften and be less starchy. Strapped for time? Let the beans sit in boiled water for 1 hour.

- If you would like to soften the recipe by bringing in milder flavors, then think about replacing the Italian sausage with a sweet sausage and adding some red chili flakes while cooking. Use spinach instead of kale and go without the beans.

Lentil Soup

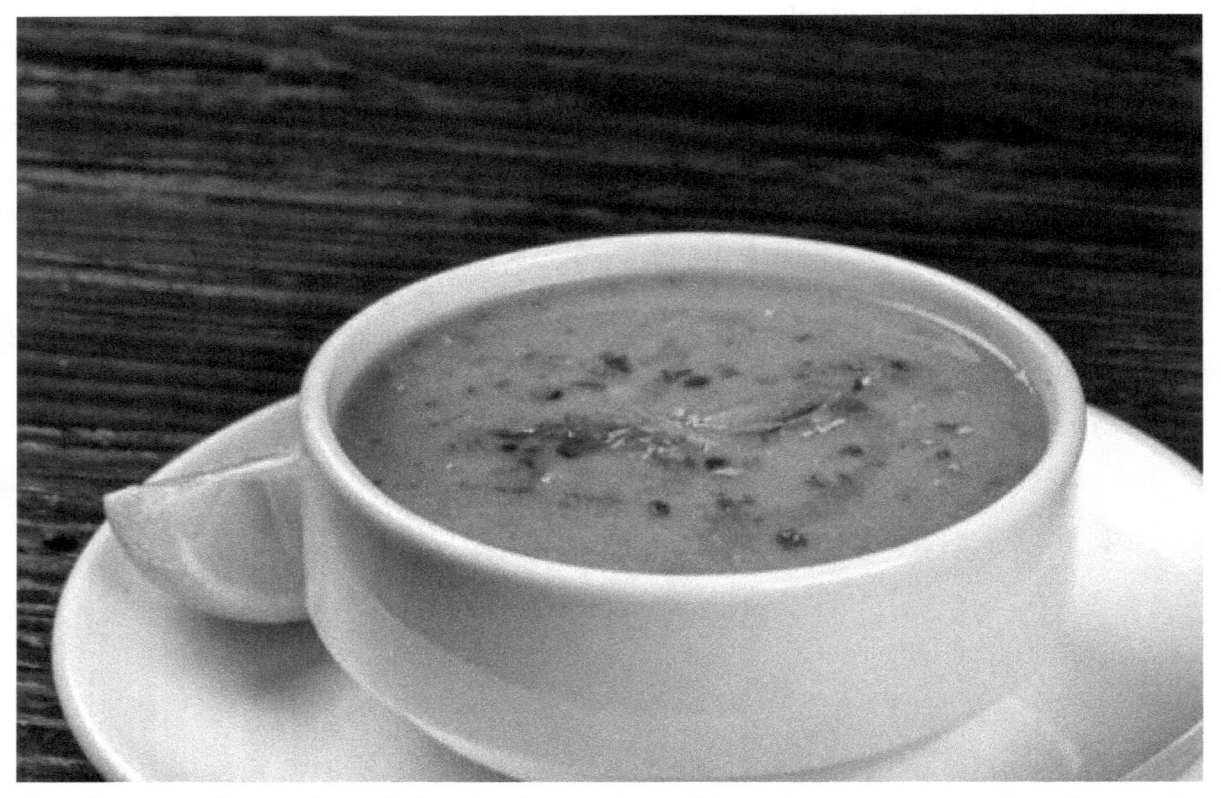

On the table you will see a classic Italian lentil soup that will happily surprise you with its flavors of tanginess and meatiness, with the added bonus of being completely vegan and gluten-free.

This is a healthy and appetizing lunch that can be reheated for a couple of days.

Total: 55 minutes

Prep Time: 15 minutes

Cooking Time: 40 minutes

Serving Size: 8 servings

Ingredients	Measurements
Lentils	1 cup
Carrots	1 cup
White onion	2 cups
Celery	1 cup
Collard greens	2 cups
Fire-roasted tomatoes	15 oz
Garlic	4 cloves
Dried thyme	¼ tsp
Red pepper flakes	¼ tsp
Dried bay leaves	2
Olive oil	2 tbsp
Vegetable stock	7 cups
Salt and pepper	Pinch

<u>Directions</u>:

1. Grab a large saucepan and add some olive oil to medium heat, inserting your peeled and diced onion, carrots, and celery. Let them sauté for around 6 minutes before adding in your minced garlic to brown for another 2 minutes.
2. Now you can add in the stock and your can of diced tomatoes, the rinsed lentils, thyme, bay leaves, red pepper flakes, and salt and pepper. Cook until it starts simmering.
3. Reduce the heat to a medium to low and cover with a lid. Let this simmer for another 30 minutes, stirring occasionally.
4. Once the lentils are tender, add in your washed collard greens and stir in for 5 minutes while also removing the bay leaves. Then serve with your choice of garnish.

<u>Nifty Tips</u>:

• If you want more meatiness to the flavor of the dish, add in chicken stock instead of vegetable stock and grate some parmesan cheese on top.

• Refrigerate for approximately 3 days in a container.

• You can use either green, red, or brown lentils.

• If you can't find a brand of fire-roasted tomatoes, just use a standard peeled and diced tomato brand.

Chickpea Soup

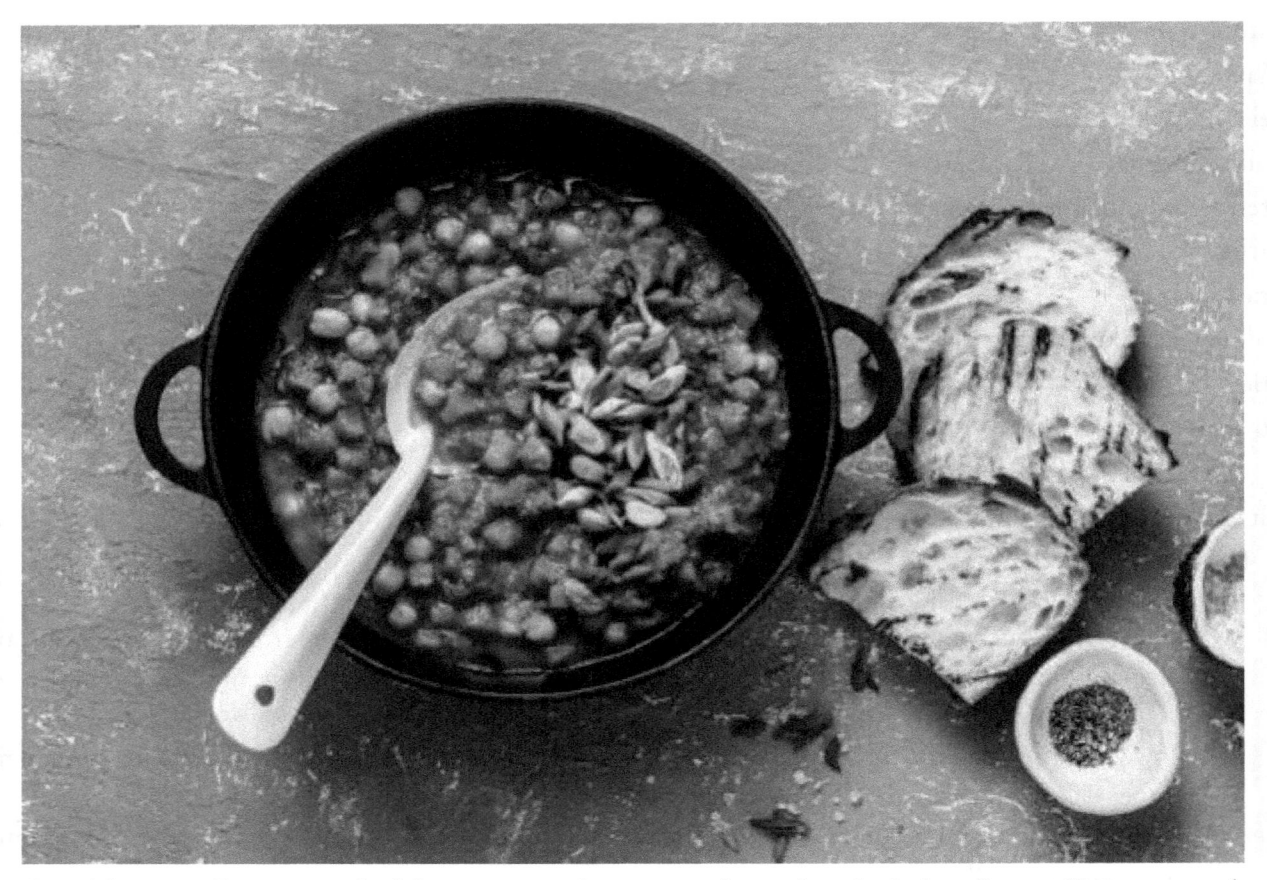

On the table you will see a wonderful soup recipe that is as traditional as the Italian flag itself. *Pasta e ceci* (pasta and chickpeas) is the basic chickpea soup that is elevated to new heights by its inclusion of short-cut pasta and parmesan rinds.

An old family favorite on fall or winter evenings, this is a healthy and generous soup.

Total: 30 minutes
Prep Time: 5 minutes
Cooking Time: 25 minutes
Serving Size: 4 servings

Ingredients	Measurements
Short cut pasta	⅓ cup
Parmesan rinds	3 rinds
Chickpeas	15 oz (1 can)
Vegetable broth	4 cups
Fire-roasted tomatoes	28 oz (2 cans)
Tomato paste	2 tbsp
Onion	1
Kale	bunch
Fresh basil	½ cup
Garlic	4 cloves
Dried oregano	½ tsp
Dried thyme	½ tsp
Red pepper flakes	2 pinches
Olive oil	2 tbsp
Salt and pepper	Pinch

Directions:

1. Let us begin by sautéing in a large pot the peeled and diced onion until translucent. Then add in your minced garlic and tomato paste, stirring for another 2 minutes.
2. Next you will add in your vegetable broth and the washed and drained chickpeas, followed by the diced tomatoes, chopped basil, thyme, oregano, and red pepper flakes. Drop in your parmesan rinds and sprinkle with some salt and pepper. Let this simmer on medium to low heat for 10 minutes.
3. Finally add in your dry pasta till cooked al dente and drop in your fresh kale. Serve with some grated parmesan.

Nifty Tips:

• If you wish to use grated parmesan instead of rinds, that works great too. Make it a ¼ cup.

• To make the simplest of vegetable broths, add your basic vegetable cuts and some herbs into boiling water for at least an hour. Sift solids out and there you go! This can be frozen and used over and over again.

• You can use standard kale for this recipe, but keep an eye out for Tuscan kale at your local vegetable markets. It holds a lot more flavor and brings that traditional sense to the meal.

Wedding Soup

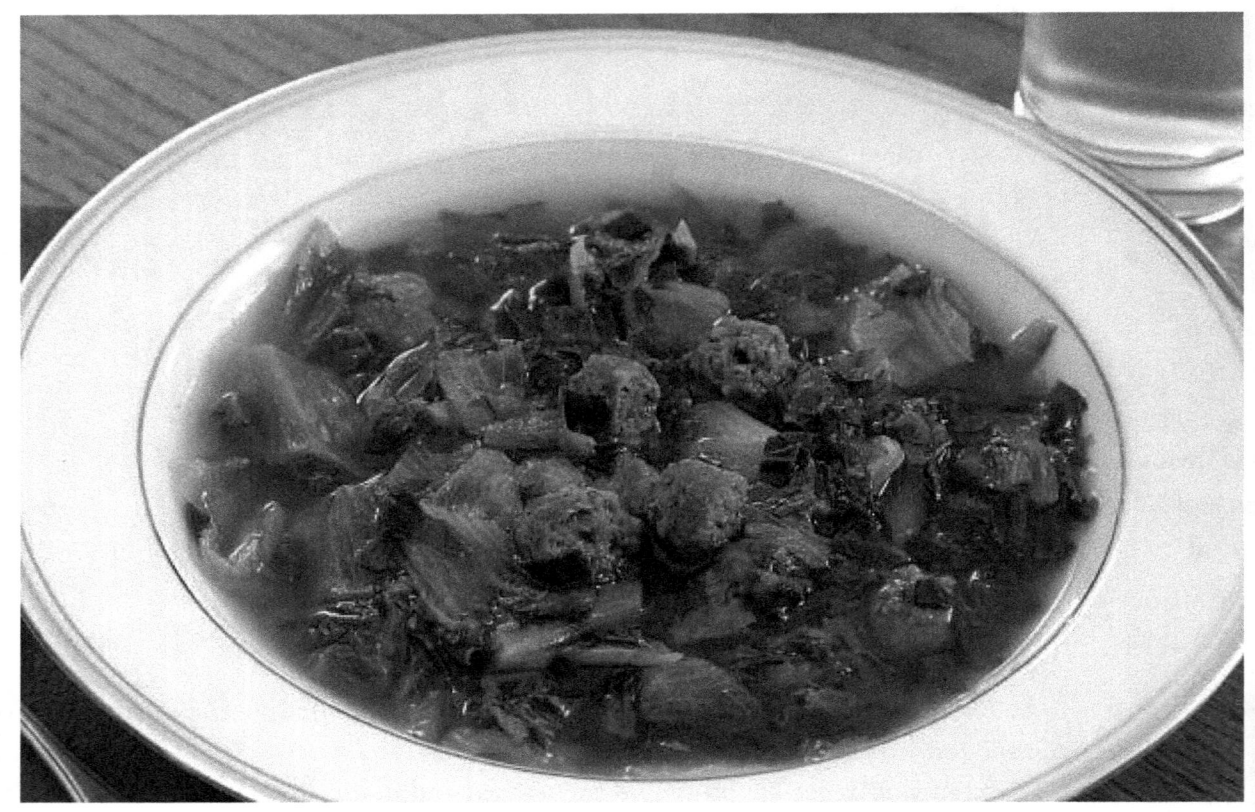

On the table you will see a pot filled with a rich broth and within a lovely variety of colors and textures. Juicy meatballs along with the kale and pasta bites make this a real combination made in heaven, like any good marriage!

This truly is a wedding of flavors coming together to bring happiness to your life.

Total: 1 hour and 20 minutes

Prep Time: 50 minutes

Cooking Time: 30 minutes

Serving Size: 8 servings

Ingredients	Measurements
Chicken stock	6 cups
Beef stock	2 cups
Ground beef	¾ lb
Italian sausage	½ lb
Egg	1 large
Seasoned breadcrumbs	⅓ cup
Parmesan	½ cup
Carrots	2
Celery	2
Onion	1
Short cut pasta	1 cup
Dry white wine	½ cup
Fresh spinach	4 oz
Fresh sage	2 tsp
Fresh chives	3 tbsp
Garlic	2 cloves
Bay leaf	1
Olive oil	2 tbsp
Water	2 cups
Salt	1 tsp

Directions:

1. Begin by preheating the oven to 350 °F (180 °C). Then start preparing the meatballs by grabbing a large mixing bowl and beating the egg, chopped sage, and chives as well as the minced garlic.
2. Throw in the ground beef, de-cased sausage, breadcrumbs, grated parmesan cheese, and ¼ tsp of salt. Combine thoroughly and begin rolling your meatballs into tablespoon-size balls. Pop them on a lined and sprayed baking tray and bake for 18 minutes till browned and juicy. Set aside to cool.
3. Grab a large saucepan and heat up to medium heat ½ tsp of olive oil. Saute your peeled and diced carrots, celery, and onion. Let them soften and glaze for 8 minutes.
4. Then add your chicken and beef broth, water, white wine, the bay leaf, and some salt and pepper. Mix it all in.
5. Drop in your pasta and turn down to medium heat to cook for around 8 minutes until al dente. Add in your meatballs and fresh spinach and let this simmer further for 5 minutes. Serve with a touch of grated parmesan and enjoy!

Nifty Tips:

- You can use all sorts of short-cut pasta like ditalini, orecchiette, penne, or rigatoni.

Chapter 9: Pasta and Sauces

We know there are tons of different kinds of pasta and many ways you can make a tasty sauce, but I would like to bring you some beginner recipes that elevate your technique, your instinct, and your palate.

From spaghetti to gnocchi, I would like to bring you a variety of pastas to test your Italian flair along with some traditional sauces that can allow you to see the real potential of good pasta.

Spaghetti Puttanesca

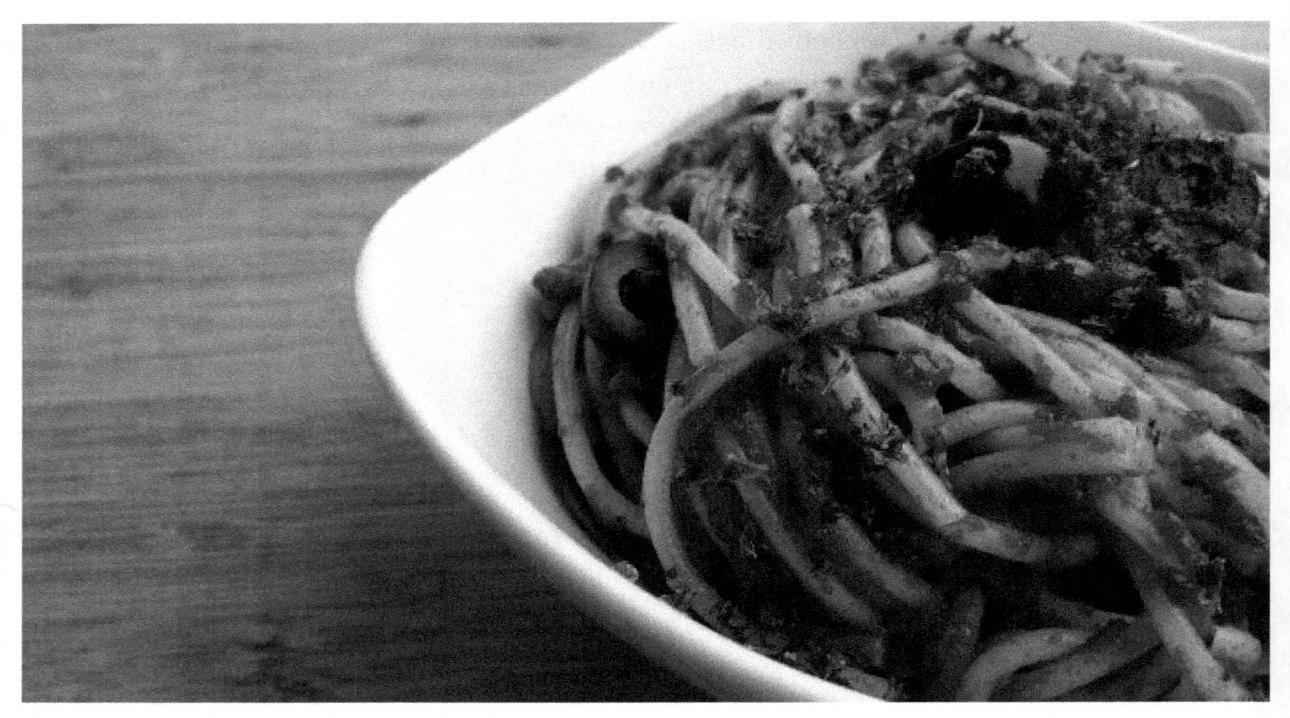

On the table you will see a dish placed, but before you see what lies within, you are met with an aroma that both invigorates and brings curiosity. As you peer at the plate you will see spaghetti topped with capers and black olives covered in a rich tomato sauce. The smell suggests that anchovies are a part of the meal, but you cannot see them. How curious!

One bite and you will be hooked. This is warm, flavorful, and decadent.

<u>Total</u>: 20 minutes

<u>Prep Time</u>: 5 minutes

<u>Cooking Time</u>: 15 minutes

<u>Serving Size</u>: 3 servings

Ingredients	Measurements
Dried spaghetti	8 oz
Anchovy filets	6
Capers	¼ cup
Black olives	¼ cup
Whole peeled tomatoes	1 cup
Parmesan cheese	1 oz
Fresh parsley	Handful
Red pepper flakes	Pinch
Garlic	4 cloves
Olive oil	6 tbsp
Salt and pepper	Pinch

Directions:

1. Start by grabbing a medium pan and bringing it to medium heat with 4 tbsp of olive oil. Add in minced garlic, finely chopped anchovy filets, and your red pepper flakes. Saute for 5 minutes until golden and aromatic, watching as the anchovies slowly dissolve.
2. Then add in your drained and chopped capers and the pitted olives. Stir occasionally at a simmer for 5 minutes then add in your tomatoes.
3. In a large pot, bring salted water to a boil, drizzling some olive oil in. Add in your pasta and cook till al dente.
4. Once it's cooked, drain your pasta but leave around 1 cup of pasta water for later use, and transfer the pasta to the saucepan. Toss up well with tongs and then add a few tbsp of pasta water into the sauce, increasing the heat to a high simmer. To loosen the sauce, add some more pasta water as you stir.
5. Finally, take the saucepan off the heat and add in your grated parmesan, chopped parsley, and remaining olive oil. Sprinkle in your salt and pepper and serve.

Nifty Tips:

- You could also add in tuna if you'd like to get a more textured sauce.

- Usually, al dente is achieved when you cook the pasta 2 minutes under the package recommendation.

Spaghetti Alla Carrettiera (Roman style)

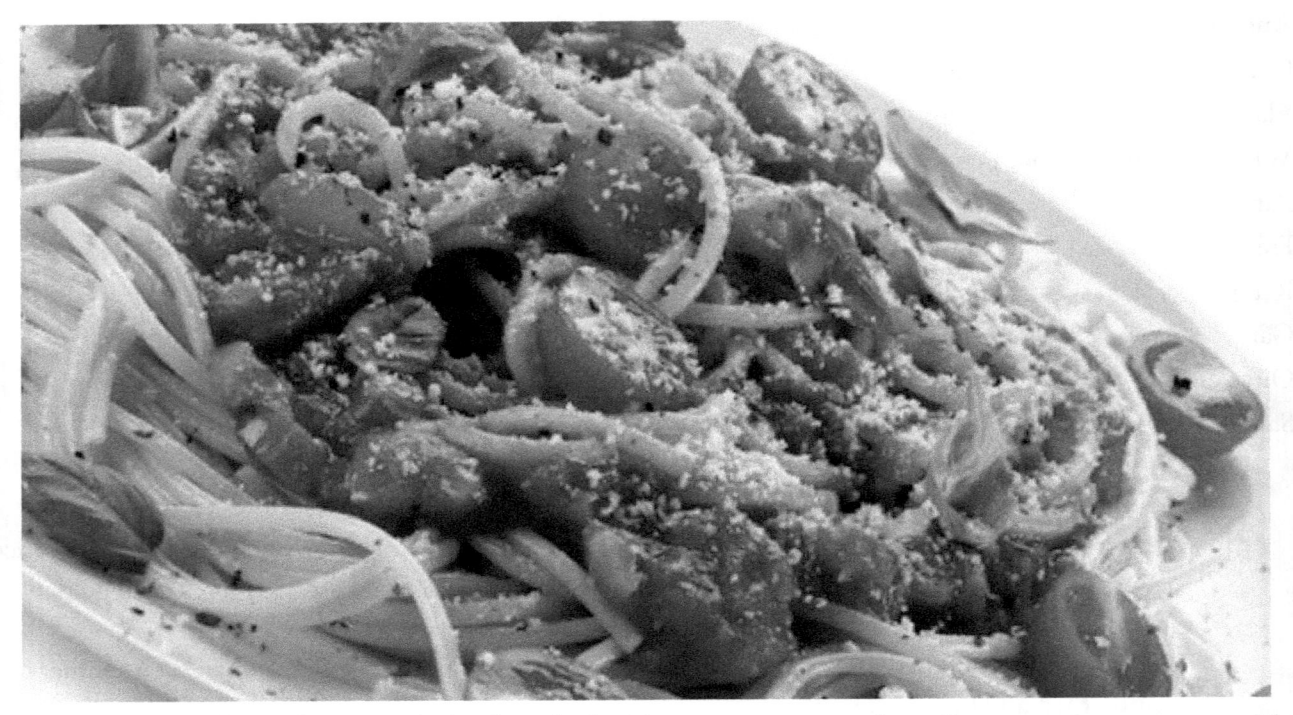

On the table you will see what can only be described as the most gorgeous plate of pasta you have ever seen. The smell of porcini mushrooms will be undeniable, along with the tinge of tuna fish and the rich tomato and tuna oil sauce.

This pasta dish can really be divine on cold winter nights or whenever you feel like indulging in extreme flavor.

<u>Total</u>: 40 minutes
<u>Prep Time</u>: 10 minutes
<u>Cooking Time</u>: 30 minutes
<u>Serving Size</u>: 4 to 6 people

Ingredients	Measurements
Dried spaghetti	1 lb
Whole peeled tomatoes	1 can (28 oz)
Fresh parsley	¼ cup
Dried porcini mushrooms	1 ½ oz (cups)
Red pepper flakes	pinch
Tuna in oil	1 can (5 oz)
Garlic	4 cloves
Olive oil	½ cup
Salt and pepper	pinch

<u>Directions</u>:

1. Let us begin by rehydrating the porcini mushrooms in a bowl of boiling water for 20 minutes. Then drain the mushrooms and put them aside, keeping ¼ cup of mushroom water for later use.
2. In a large pot, bring together your ¼ cup of olive oil and minced garlic. Sprinkle in your red pepper flakes and 1 tbsp of chopped parsley and at medium heat, and cook for 3 minutes.
3. Now take your drained mushrooms and add them to the pot of oil. Saute for 1 minute.
4. Add in your mushroom water and tomatoes then add 2 tbsp of oil from the tuna can and bring to a simmer with some salt and pepper.
5. Bring a medium pot of salted and oiled water to a boil, and cook the spaghetti till al dente.
6. Now take your drained tuna and flake it off into the sauce; toss in your cooked spaghetti along with your ¼ cup of pasta water.
7. Cook for a further 3 minutes till the sauce has coated the pasta sufficiently and has combined well. Then add in your remaining olive oil and chopped parsley. Combine and serve.

Spaghetti Aglio e Olio (Garlic and Olive oil)

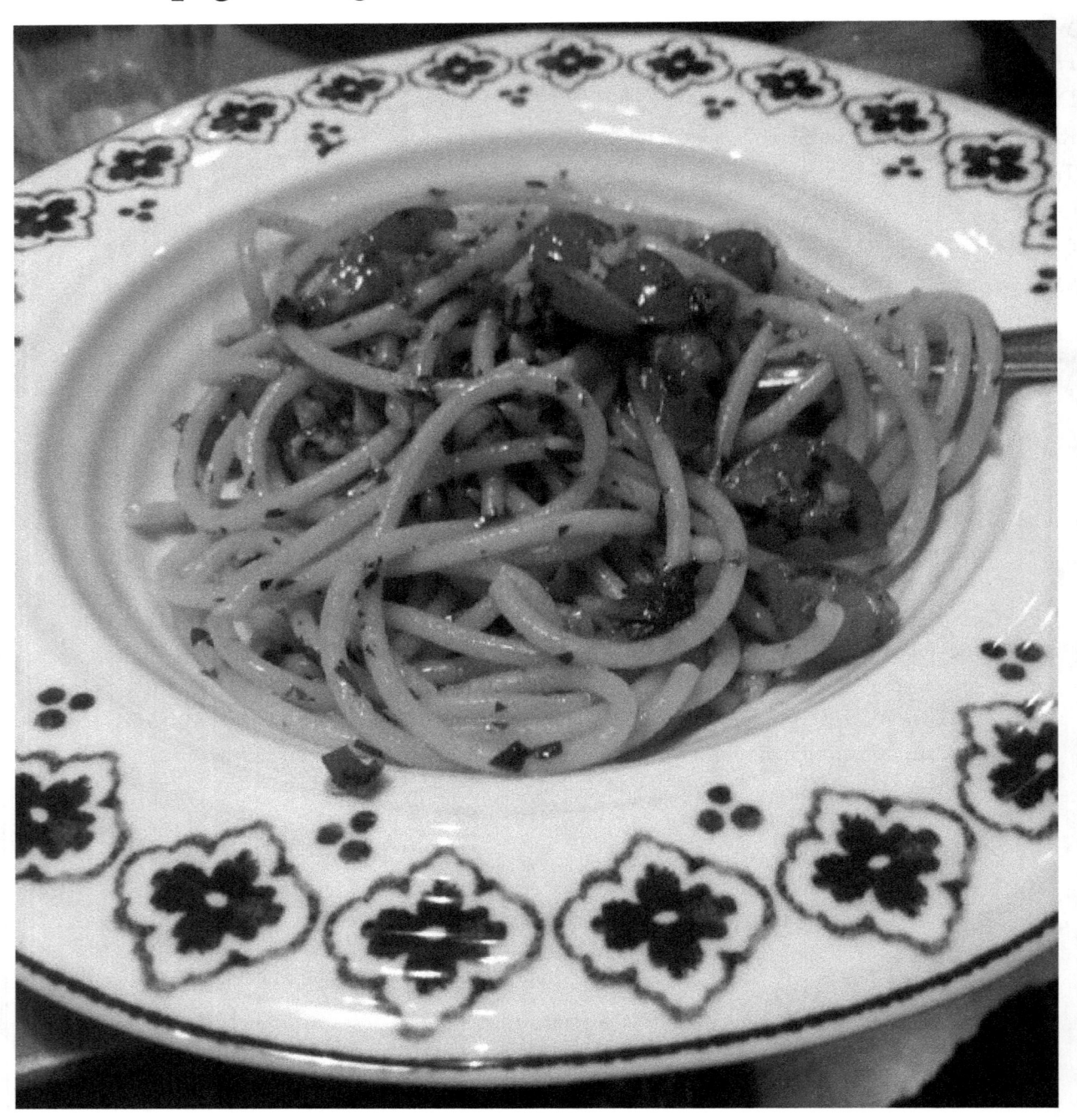

On the table you will see a plate of spaghetti, and from afar it could be any old simple bowl of spaghetti. But as you smell and taste the garlic, olive oil, and the subtle red pepper you can only be surprised at how easy it is to bring it together!

Total Cooking Time: 10 minutes

<u>Serving Size</u>: 4 servings

Ingredients	Measurements
Dried spaghetti	1 lb (16 oz)
Fresh parsley	Pinch
Red pepper flakes	Pinch
Garlic	4 cloves
Olive oil	½ cup
Salt and pepper	Pinch

<u>Directions</u>:

1. Begin by boiling your salted water for the spaghetti in a medium pot, cook al dente, and keep the pasta water.
2. In a large pan, add in 6 tbsp of olive oil and the thinly sliced garlic, followed by the red pepper flakes. Allow this to brown for 5 minutes
3. Take your drained pasta and drop it in the hot oil pan, with a cup of your pasta water. Combine with vigor to emulsify the oil with the pasta.
4. Serve with a sprinkle of parsley and a drizzle of olive oil once you have taken it off the heat.

Sage and Butter Gnocchi

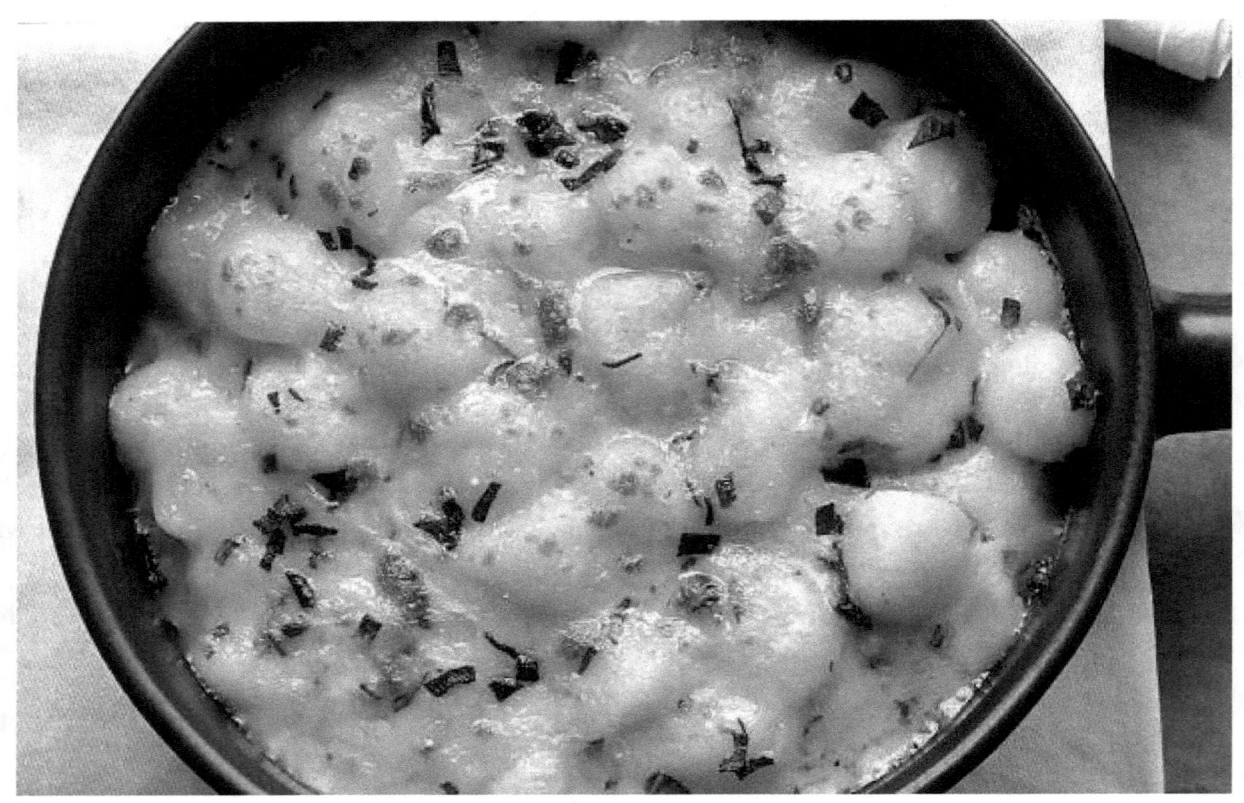

On the table you will see a divine-looking bowl of soft and round gnocchi covered in a sweet and aromatic sauce. The smell of cooked sage swimming in butter is just the right flavor for the robust but light potato gnocchi.

Dive in and enjoy with gusto! This is great for family lunches and dinners.

Total: 1 hour 45 minutes
Prep Time: 45 minutes
Cooking Time: 60 minutes
Serving Size: 4 servings

Ingredients	Measurements
AP flour	¾ cup
Russet potatoes	3 lb
Eggs	3
Fresh sage	15 leaves
Parmesan	Grating
Unsalted butter	4 oz
Salt and pepper	pinch

Special Equipment:

- Food mill
- Slotted spoon
- Bench scraper

Directions:

1. Let us start by preheating the oven to 450 °F (230 °C).
2. Next, scrub and clean your potatoes, poke them evenly with a sharp knife, and place them on your lined baking tray with sprinkled salt. Bake for 45 minutes till soft.
3. Then take your cooled potatoes and halve them lengthwise; grab a large spoon and scoop out as much potato flesh as you can into a bowl.
4. Now process the potato flesh by pressing it through the food mill in its finest filter, onto a clean surface. To allow it to cool more efficiently, spread out evenly.
5. Take your eggs, and separate the yolks. Whisk the yolks thoroughly and add them over the spread-out potato mash.
6. Sift about ½ cup of AP flour over the mash and then take your bench scraper and cut in the potato, flour, and egg until well combined.
7. Gather up all the potato mix and create a rough ball then press the ball flat, cut in half with your bench scraper, and flatten once more.
8. Take your other ¼ cup of flour and sift over the mixture, then fold gently and press down until a consistent and smooth dough.
9. On a floured surface, shape the dough into a log. Slice 1 inch portions rolled into ½ inch thick strings. Now cut those strings into 1 inch segments. Once all strings are created, transfer to a lined baking sheet.
10. Bring a large pot of salted water to a boil and then bring a skillet to a medium to high temperature with butter and sage. Fry until butter is lightly golden and then remove from heat.
11. Transfer gnocchi to boiling water. Avoid sticking by stirring gently with the slotted spoon. Wait for the gnocchi to start floating and after about 20 seconds give one a taste. It must not taste like flour.
12. Next, you will directly transfer the gnocchi into the sage butter pan over medium heat. Add a little gnocchi water to even the texture of the sauce and toss well until the sauce is creamy.
13. Serve with grated parmesan cheese.

Nifty Tips:

- When folding and pressing the mash, try not to smear the dough as this could break the bond.

Ricotta Gnocchi With Asparagus and Prosciutto

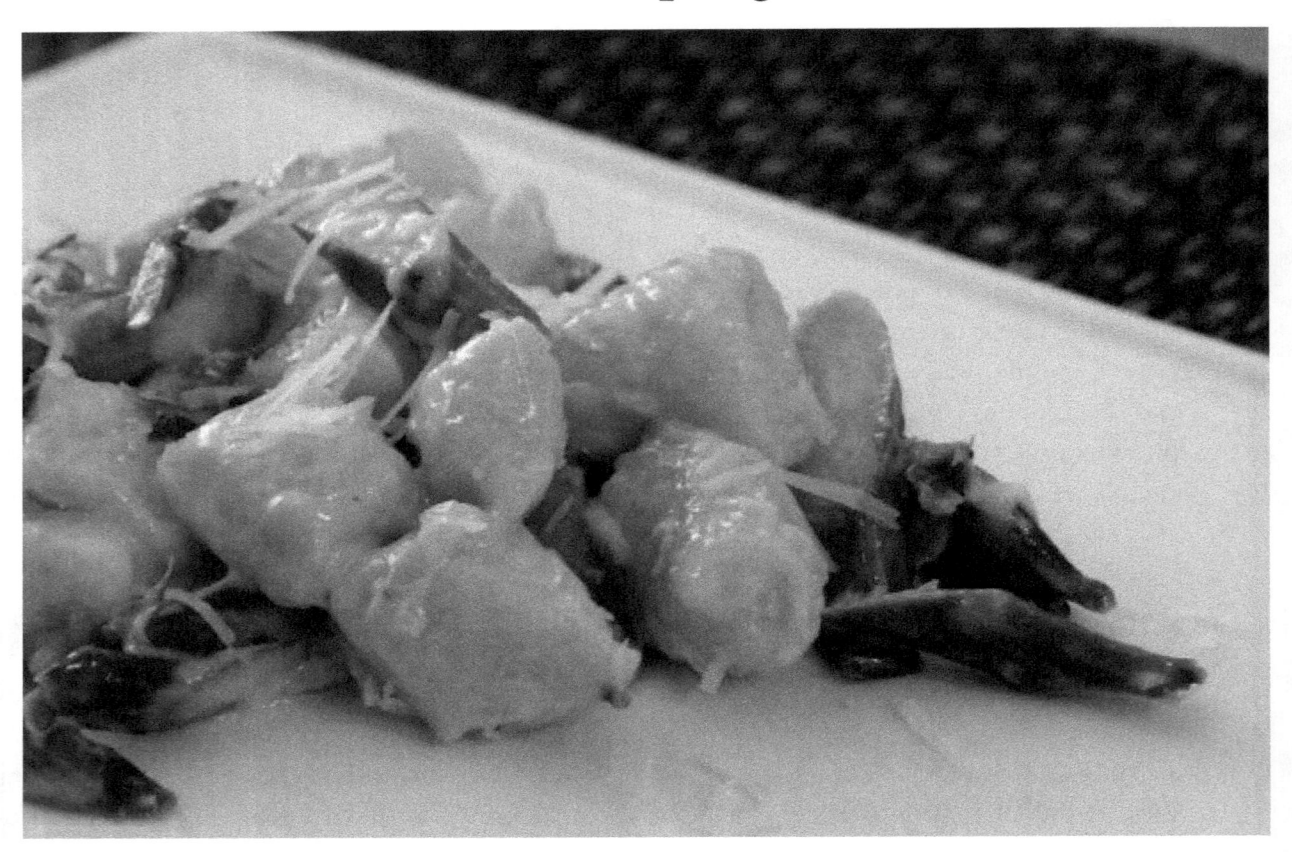

On the table you will see a divine-looking bowl of soft and round gnocchi covered in a soft white sauce. And what is that there? Asparagus pieces, yes, and some prosciutto pieces too. The colorful arrangement on the plate is beautiful and looks delicious.

Tuck in! See what flavors can be found with the fresh and the salty.

Total: 20 minutes

Prep Time: 10 minutes

Cooking Time: 10 minutes

Serving Size: 3 to 4 servings

Ingredients	Measurements
Ricotta gnocchi	500g (2 cups + 1 tbsp)
Asparagus	1 lb
Fresh chives	2 tbsp
Parmesan	2 oz
Prosciutto	4 oz
Heavy cream	1 cup
Garlic	2 cloves
Scallions (spring onion)	¼ cup
Olive oil	1 tbsp
Lemon	1
Salt and pepper	pinch

Directions:

1. Start by boiling a large pot of salted water. Heat up a pan with olive oil. In the pan, add your prosciutto slices and cook for around 2 minutes. Add the thinly sliced scallions and allow this to saute for 1 minute.
2. Cut your asparagus into 1 ½ inch sections and toss in, cooking for another 2 minutes until the asparagus turns tender and vibrant green.
3. Now you will add in your heavy cream and half of your grated parmesan. Stir well until smooth and creamy for 4 minutes, sprinkling in some salt and pepper for taste.
4. Drop your gnocchi into the boiling water, letting each batch cook for 3 minutes until they start floating. Wait 20 seconds and then remove and drain. Keep a ¼ cup of gnocchi water for later.
5. In the saucepan, add in your gnocchi, lemon zest, lemon juice, chopped chives, and 2 tbsp of gnocchi water. Let this come to a hard boil, adding more gnocchi water until the desired consistency is reached.
6. Serve hot and sprinkle with some lemon zest and the remaining parmesan cheese.

Nifty Tips:

- Follow the recipe in Chapter 7 to make ricotta gnocchi.

Creamy Mushroom Pasta

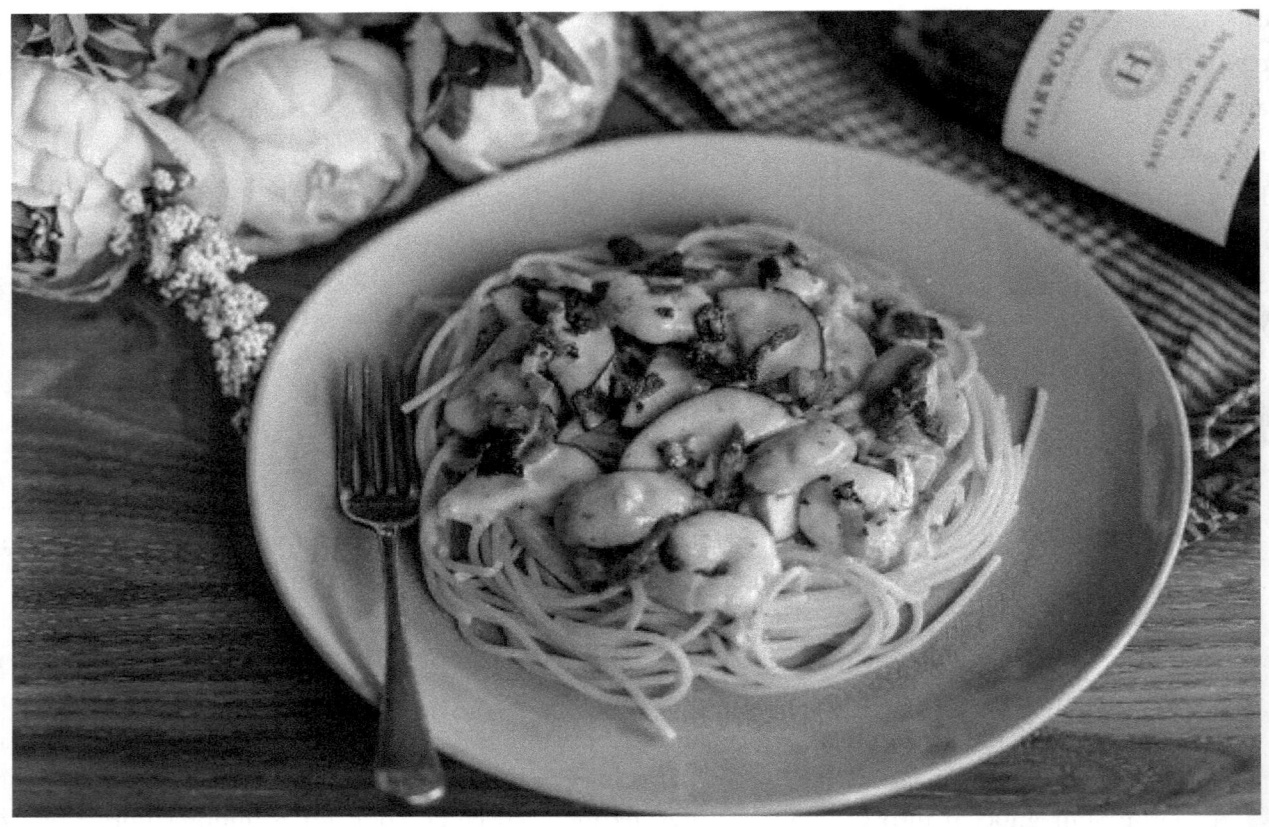

On the table you will see a bowl of different-looking pasta. These short-cut and tubular pastas work wonders with the sauce, as it fills the interior of the pasta and allows you to get more sauce with every bite. Creamy with the earthy taste of mushrooms, this dish is just a winner.

   Total: 40 minutes
   Prep Time: 10 minutes
   Cooking Time: 30 minutes
   Serving Size: 4 servings

Ingredients	Measurements
Short cut pasta	1 lb
Mixed mushroom	1 ½ lb
Chicken stock	1 cup
Powdered gelatine	1 ½ tsp
Shallots	¾ cup
Dry white wine	½ cup
Fresh thyme	2 tbsp
Fresh parsley	¼ cup
Garlic	2 cloves
Unsalted butter	3 oz
Olive oil	2 tbsp
Parmesan	1 cup
Fish sauce	1 tsp
Salt and pepper	pinch

<u>Directions</u>:

1. Let us begin by taking our chicken stock, pouring it into a small bowl and sprinkling the powdered gelatine over the surface. Set aside.
2. Over medium to high heat, take your pan and add in olive oil. Once hot, add in your torn mushrooms and salt and pepper. Allow the mushrooms to brown in oil for 15 minutes.
3. Now we can add in the peeled and finely minced shallots, the chopped thyme leaves, and the minced garlic. Keep this cooking for 2 minutes until soft.
4. Pour in your white wine and let simmer. Use a wooden spoon to scrape any sticky bits from the skillet.
5. Add in your chicken stock, season with salt and pepper, and bring to a simmer.
6. Now reduce the heat and add in your fish sauce. Thicken the sauce for about 5 minutes and turn off the heat.
7. Place your pasta in a pot of boiling salt water until it's just under al dente. Strain the pasta and retain 1 cup of pasta water.
8. Transfer the pasta to the skillet and toss well to incorporate. Cook for 2 minutes and then add in your pasta water slowly.
9. Add in your butter until melted and remove from heat. Sprinkle on ¾ cup of grated parmesan and chopped parsley. Stir vigorously to combine. Serve with a sprinkle of the remaining parmesan.

<u>Nifty Tips</u>:

- You can use shitake, oyster, maitake, or beech mushroom to name a few. Instead of slicing the mushrooms, try tearing them apart with your fingers to increase earthy flavor.

Four-Cheese Pasta

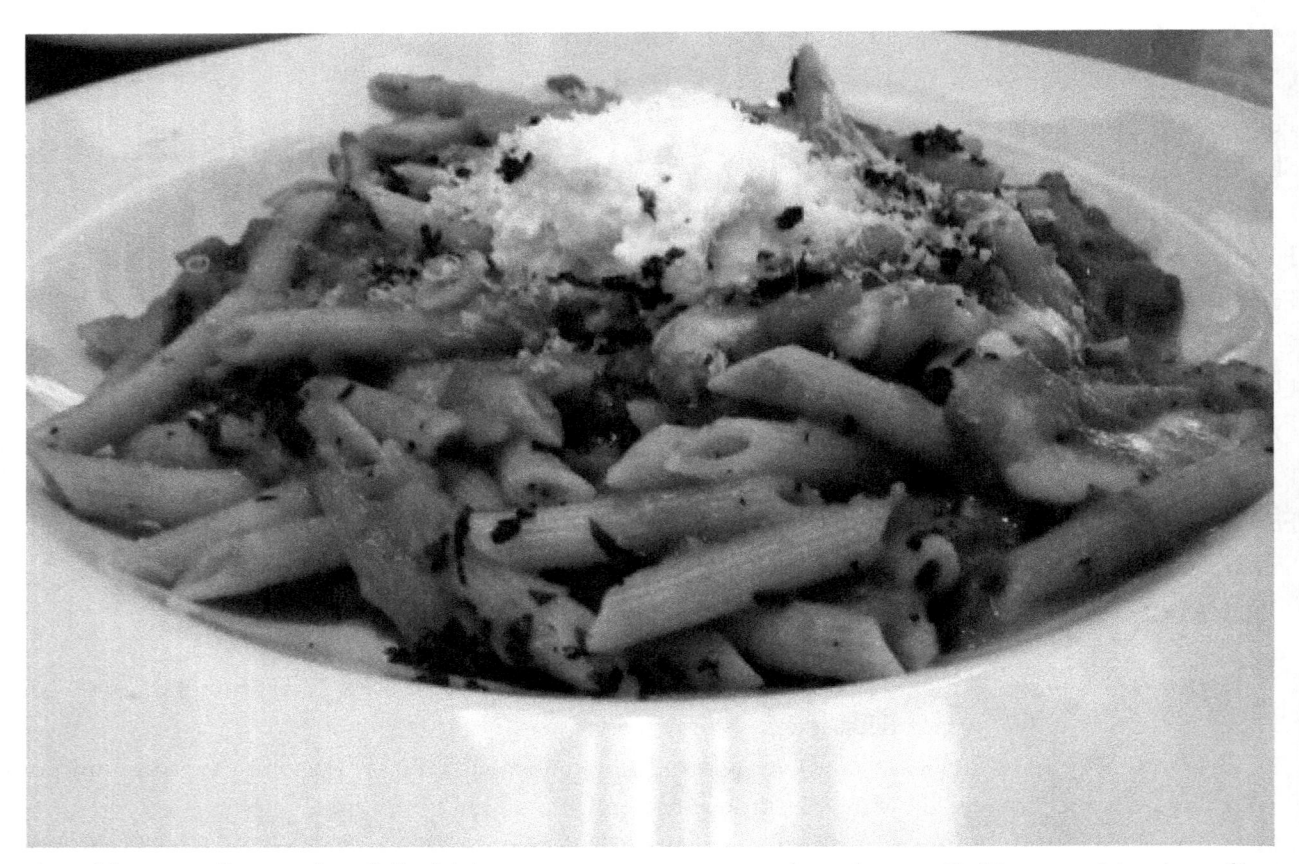

On the table you will see a plate full of delicious penne pasta covered in what smells like a combination of heaven and paradise. The aroma of various cheeses will fill your senses.

This four-cheese pasta is a must for parties and family gatherings.

<u>Total</u>: 35 minutes
<u>Prep Time</u>: 10 minutes
<u>Cooking Time</u>: 25 minutes
<u>Serving Size</u>: 4 servings

Ingredients	Measurements
Penne or fusilli pasta	1 lb
Heavy cream	1 cup
Parmesan cheese	1 ½ oz
Taleggio cheese	3 oz
Fontina cheese	3 oz
Gorgonzola cheese	3 oz
Fresh thyme	3 tbsp (1 sprig)
Garlic	1 clove
Olive oil	1 tbsp
Salt	Pinch
Ground black pepper	½ tsp

Directions:

1. Begin by heating up your heavy cream, whole thyme sprigs, lightly ruptured garlic clove, and black pepper at medium heat in a medium saucepan till it begins simmering. Scrape the bottom of the pan with a wooden spoon every now and then to prevent burning. Remove from heat, let it steep for 5 minutes and then discard the garlic and thyme.
2. Return the cream to low heat, adding in your chopped taleggio cheese. Make sure to gently whisk it all together till evenly melted.
3. Now add in your grated Fontina, still whisking until a smooth consistency develops. Then add the finely grated parmesan. Keep at a very low simmer.
4. Next you will drop your pasta into a boiling pot of salted water until just al dente. Then strain and add it to the saucepan to be mixed well with the cheese sauce, always keeping 1 cup of pasta water nearby to add in if too thick.
5. Remove the saucepan from the heat and stir in your broken and chunky gorgonzola pieces. Serve immediately.

Nifty Tips:

- If you want a chunkier sauce, leave the gorgonzola for the guests to add to their plates so it does not melt too soon.

- Try all sorts of different hard cheeses, but stay away from dense yellow cheeses like gouda and stringy cheeses like mozzarella.

Pasta alla Norma (Sicilian style)

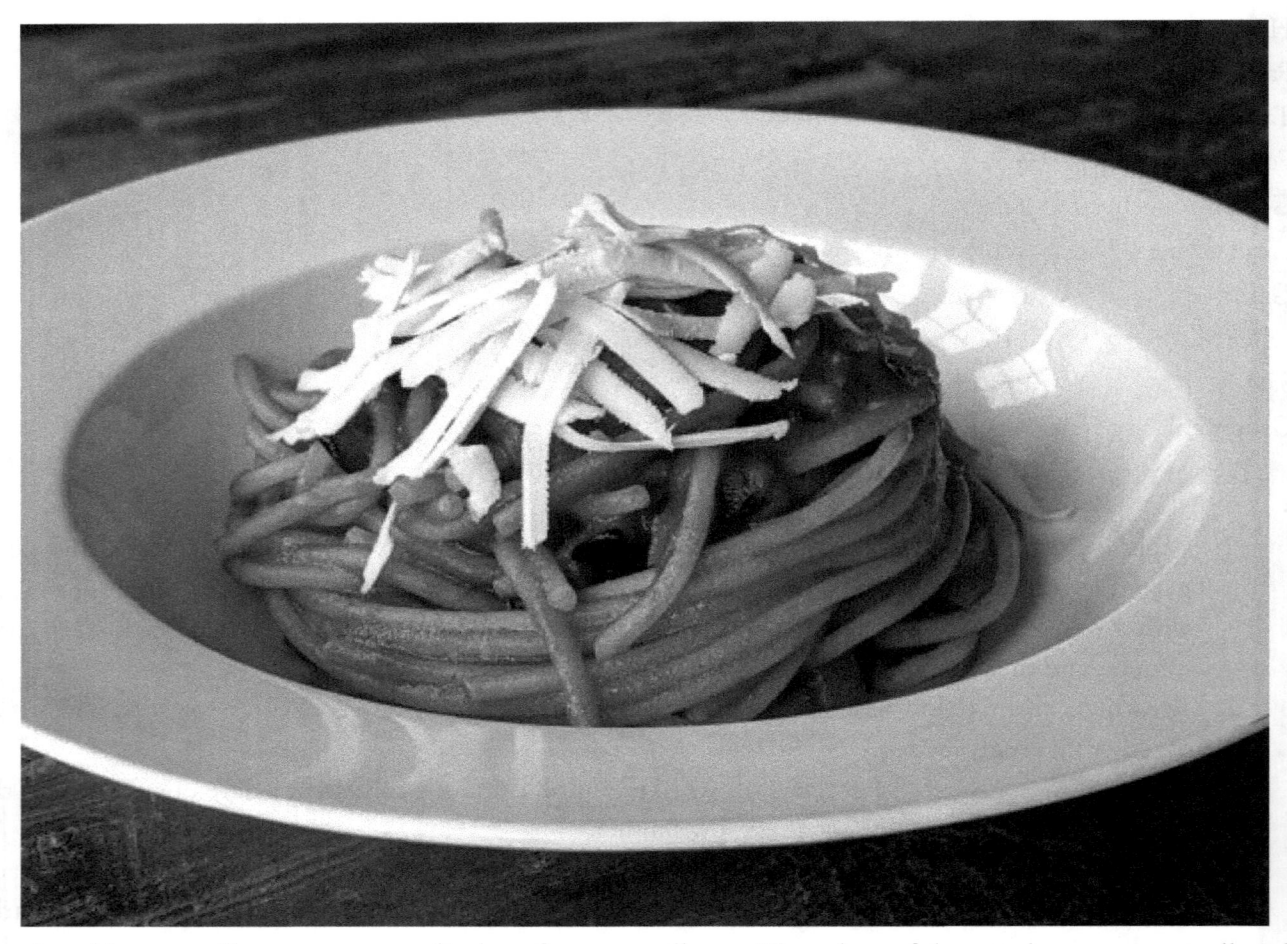

On the table, you will see a gorgeous display of pasta excellency. The colors of the eggplant contrast well with the fresh green basil and the white salted ricotta. The unmistakable taste of cooked eggplant brings its meatiness, and the freshness of the tomato is to die for.

There is a busyness to this dish that just asks to be devoured but savored.

Total: 50 minutes

Prep Time: 30 minutes

Cooking Time: 20 minutes

Serving Size: 4 servings

Ingredients	Measurements
Rigatoni or penne pasta	1 lb
Salted ricotta	2 oz
Eggplants	¾ lb
Fresh basil	12 leaves
Whole peeled tomatoes	28 oz
Tomato paste	2 tbsp
Olive oil	6 tbsp
Red pepper flakes	¼ tsp
Dried oregano	1 tbsp
Garlic	3 cloves
Salt and pepper	Pinch

Special Equipment:

- Skillet

Directions:

1. Begin by cleaning and cutting your eggplants. Split each eggplant lengthwise, then slice each half into ½ inch slices.
2. Heat up your medium skillet over medium heat and drizzle in 2 tbsp olive oil until hot. Then place your eggplant slices evenly at the base of the skillet in one layer, without overpacking. Sprinkle the layer with salt and then proceed to brown each side evenly for around 10 minutes. Set aside on paper towels to drain, and repeat the process until all batches are done, making sure you replenish the olive oil as you go.
3. In the same skillet, increase the heat to medium-high, placing your minced garlic, oregano, and red pepper flakes into the remaining olive oil. Let this cook for only 30 seconds to avoid browning the garlic.
4. Add in your tomato paste and combine until you start to see the paste frying. Throw in your hand crushed whole tomatoes, reducing the heat and stirring well for 10 minutes until the sauce thickens nicely.
5. Cook your pasta in boiling salted water till just al dente and always keep some of the pasta water. Drain the pasta and toss it into the skillet, adding in the pasta water to reduce thickness. Follow this with your fried eggplant slices and stir to combine flavors well.
6. Lastly, add in your broken up salted ricotta pieces and a drizzle of olive oil, then serve immediately.

Pesto alla Trapanese (Sicilian Style Almonds and Tomato)

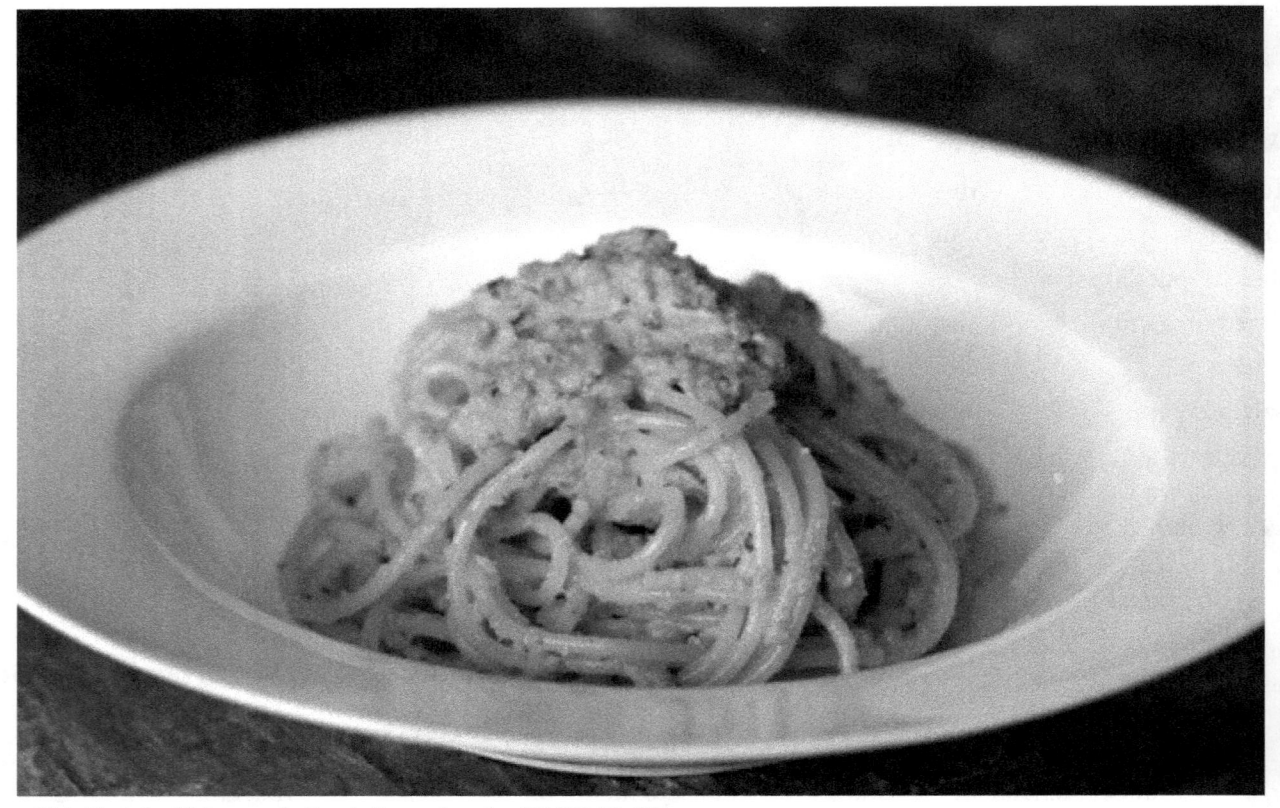

This Photo by Unknown Author is licensed under CC BY-SA-NC

On the table, you will see a bowl of warm and inviting pasta. It is covered with various toppings, all infusing each other in divine combinations. The toasted almonds, the pecorino cheese, and the fresh mint make complete sense when you are biting into it.

Total: 20 minutes
Prep Time: 10 minutes
Cooking Time: 10 minutes
Serving Size: 4 people

Ingredients	Measurements
Linguini pasta	1 lb
Plum tomatoes	1 lb
Fresh mint	4 leaves
Fresh basil	35 large leaves
Pecorino	3 ½ oz
Roasted and blanched almonds	2 oz
Olive oil	¼ cup
Garlic	3 cloves
Salt and pepper	pinch

<u>Special Equipment</u>:

- Large mortar and pestle

<u>Directions</u>:

1. Begin by crushing the garlic and a pinch of salt in the mortar and pestle until a thick paste shows. Add your almonds and beat further. Add your whole basil and mint leaves while still consistently crushing. Then finally add in your grated pecorino cheese and your tomatoes and the olive oil to create a thick sauce.
2. Take about ⅔ of that sauce and place it in a large serving bowl.
3. Cook your pasta in a large boiling pot of salted water for 10 minutes until just al dente. Strain and transfer the pasta on top of the sauce in the serving bowl, adding some of the kept pasta water to dilute the sauce if needed.
4. Toss well and serve with a big dollop of the remaining sauce on each portion with some grated cheese as desired.

<u>Nifty Tips</u>:

- You can easily use a food processor for step 1.

Chapter 10: Risotto

What more can one say about risotto other than it is an incredibly unique dish. Someone once tried to explain risotto to me by describing it as, "Oh you know, that sticky and thick rice dish." Yes, that delicious and decadent sticky rice dish that when done well, can be as addictive as hell.

This filling and rich meal can be experimented with in various flavors and notes. The rice is always the same and the basic method for preparing and rehydrating is there, but each recipe brings along a signature style and presentation.

Let's take a look at a few recipes that I really consider to be a basic foundation for any beginner.

Perfect Risotto

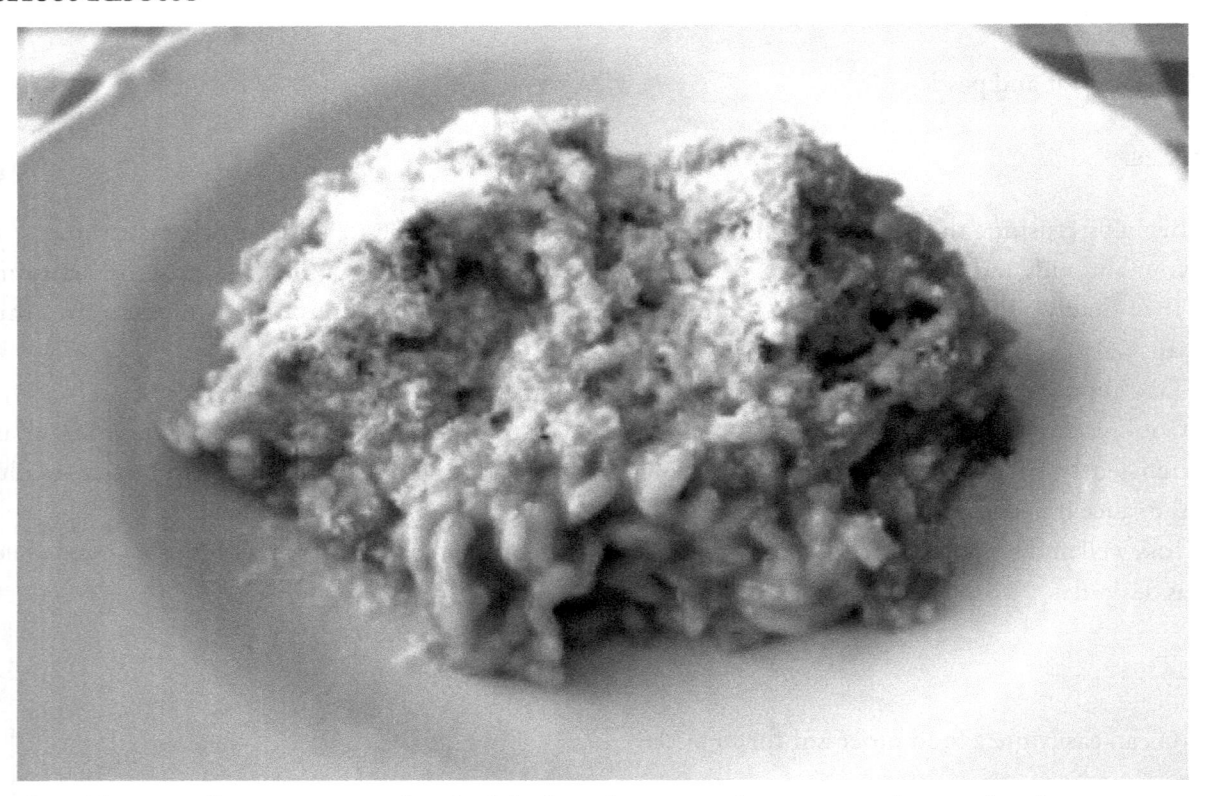

On the table you will see a steaming bowl of thick sticky risotto. It is creamy white and makes your mouth water with its heavy infusion of cheese, cream, and butter. As arguably the most comforting comfort food out there, this risotto can turn the dullest day bright!

Total: 30 minutes

Prep Time: 15 minutes

Cooking Time: 15 minutes

Serving Size: 4 to 6 servings

Ingredients	Measurements
Risotto rice	1 ½ cups
Dry white wine	1 cup
Parmesan cheese	3 oz
Heavy cream	¾ cup
Shallots	2
Garlic	2 cloves
Chicken stock	4 cups
Salted butter	2 tbsp
Olive oil	2 tbsp
Salt and pepper	pinch

<u>Directions</u>:

1. Let us start by combining in a large bowl the risotto rice, the chicken stock, and the white wine. Gently whisk the rice to release the starch.
2. Now you can strain the rice into a large bowl and let it drain for 5 minutes. Keep stirring the rice as it drains, but keep the rice broth.
3. In a large skillet, over medium to high heat, mix your butter and oil. Once the foaming stops, add your drained rice, and cook the remaining liquid away.
4. As soon as the rice has a golden brown color, add the grated garlic and the finely minced shallots and simmer for about 1 minute.
5. Take your rice broth and give it a thorough stir then add it slowly into the risotto mix, keeping 1 cup set aside. Heat this up at a high temperature until simmering.
6. Stir the rice mix only once, cover it, and lower the temperature to the lowest heat. Allow this to cook for 10 minutes undisturbed.
7. Stir once again and wait for another 10 minutes until most of the liquid has been absorbed.
8. Now add in your last remaining cup of rice broth, and stir in well until creamy and thick.
9. Remove the saucepan from the heat and grate in your parmesan cheese while also folding in the heavy cream. Serve with some salt and pepper and garnish.

<u>Nifty Tips</u>:

- Risotto rice needs to be tasted as you go. Make sure that the consistency is dense, but not starchy. Think in terms of al dente risotto.

Risotto With Spring Peas, Fontina, and Ham

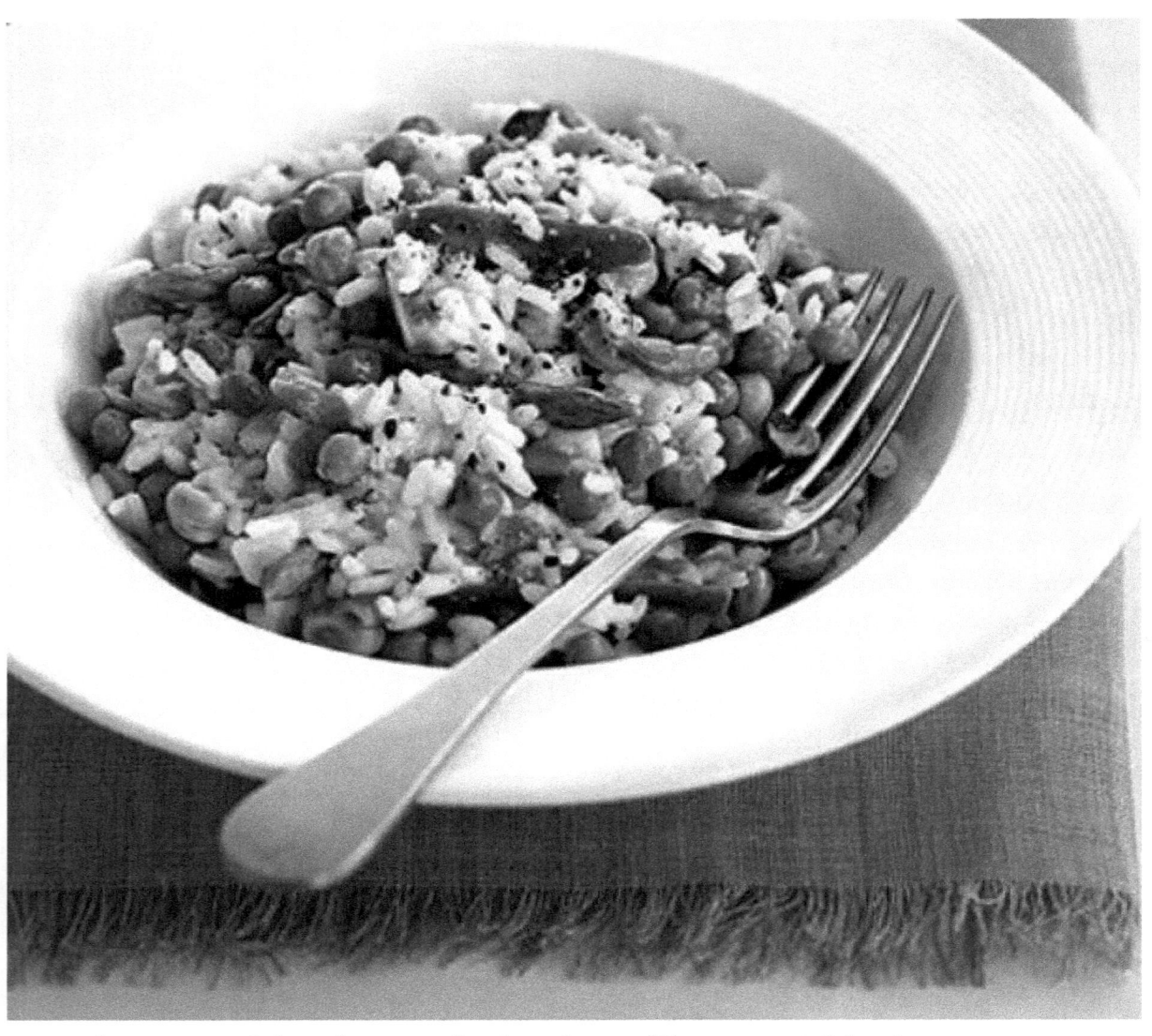

This is another stunning dish to show your family and yourself how resourceful and creative you are!

<u>Total</u>: 35 minutes

<u>Prep Time</u>: 10 minutes

<u>Cooking Time</u>: 25 minutes

<u>Serving Size</u>: 4 to 6 servings

Ingredients	Measurements
Risotto rice	1 ½ cups
Shelled baby peas	1 cup
Chicken or vegetable broth	4 cups
Dry white wine	½ cup
Ham	1 cup
Fontina cheese	1 cup
Onion	⅓ cup
Fresh basil	2 tbsp
Salted butter	4 tbsp
Olive oil	2 tbsp
Lemon	1
Salt and pepper	Pinch

Directions:

1. We shall begin by firstly heating olive oil and half the butter in a large saucepan over medium heat.
2. Add the finely chopped onion for 5 minutes until glossy.
3. Add in your risotto rice and stir until fully coated, for around 3 minutes.
4. Next, add in the white wine and continue to cook until it has been absorbed completely. Then grab 3 cups of warmed-up broth and ladle in one cup at a time until absorbed for approximately 20 minutes.
5. While adding the last cup of broth, also pop in half of your grated Fontina cheese, 1 tbsp of lemon zest, the finely diced ham, and baby peas. Sprinkle salt and pepper and mix thoroughly. This should cook for another 5 minutes.
6. Remove from heat and stir in the remainder of the cheese and butter. Once all is mixed well, serve.

Nifty Tips:

- Remember to always serve risotto on a warmed-up plate or bowl to avoid the rice congealing.

Corn Risotto in Pressure Cooker

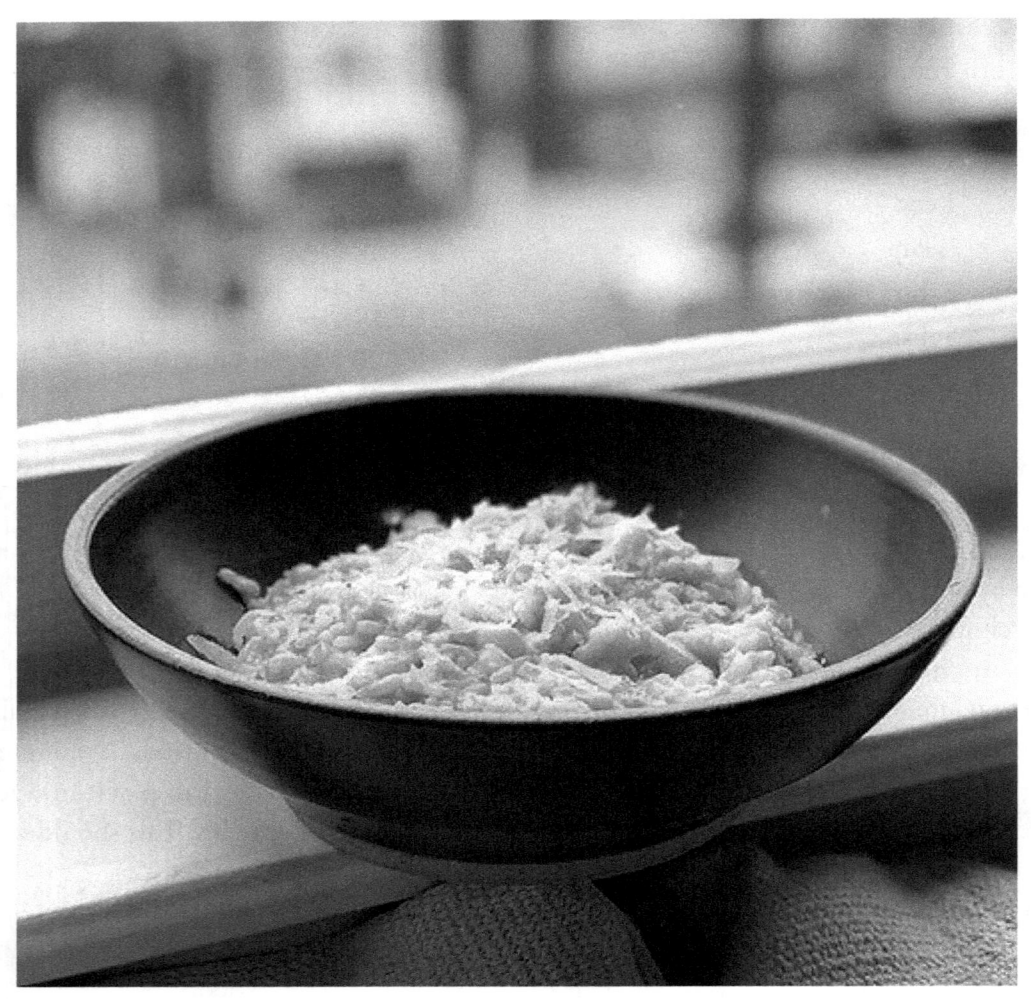

On the table you will see a gorgeous yellow gold bowl of risotto that will bring sweetness to your day. The corn carries a lot of subtle flavors that thickens and creams the risotto perfectly.

A pressure cooker is a great addition to any kitchen, no matter what cuisine you experiment with.

Total: 40 minutes
Prep Time: 20 minutes
Cooking Time: 20 minutes
Serving Size: 4 to 6 servings

Ingredients	Measurements
Risotto rice	2 cups
Corn	6 ears
Shallots	2 small (2 oz)
Dry white wine	¾ cup (6 oz)
Heavy cream	¼ cup
Chicken or vegetable stock	3 ½ cups
Bay leaf	1
Fresh thyme	3 sprigs
Unsalted butter	6 tbsp
Garlic	2 cloves
Ground turmeric	1 tsp
Parmesan cheese	½ cup
Salt and pepper	Pinch

Special Equipment:

- Pressure cooker
- Food processor or emulsifier

Directions:

1. We will start by rinsing the risotto rice in your cold stock in a medium bowl. Stir occasionally with a wooden spoon to release the starch. Then strain the rice through a fine-mesh sieve. Keep the stock for later.
2. Next you will want to de-husk your corn and trim the corn from the cobs into a small bowl. Scrape off as much starch from the cob as possible with the flat-backed knife. Make sure to keep 3 of the clean cobs for later use.
3. Now we will preheat the pressure cooker to saute heat and place 2 tbsp of butter inside to melt for 1 minute. Introduce the corn and saute for a further 2 minutes. Once all cooked and tender, remove from the pressure cooker to cool aside.
4. Again you will want to place your remaining 4 tbsp of butter into the pressure cooker for another minute to melt and foam. Next, add in the minced shallots and the minced garlic and sweat for approximately 2 minutes.
5. Now we can add the strained risotto rice to the pressure cooker for 2 minutes until toasted, followed by your white wine which will need to be reduced quite a bit. Taste it every 30 seconds until the acidic taste has evaporated, which will be after around 2 minutes.
6. Then we add in the whole bay leaf, thyme sprigs, and the stock kept from the rice. Stir and season with salt and pepper while also adding in those 3 reserved cobs, closing the lid, and cooking for 4 minutes.

7. As the risotto cooks, put half the sautéed corn along with your heavy cream and turmeric into a food processor or blender and blitz until smooth and creamy then set aside.
8. Once the risotto is cooked, you will want to depressurize the cooker by slowly releasing the pressure valve. Begin by removing the bay leaves and the thyme as well as the corn cobs, making sure to scrape any remaining liquid back into the risotto.
9. Now we can add in the corn puree and the other half of the sauteed corn, along with the grated parmesan. Create a creamy texture by stirring continuously for another 2 minutes. Serve with some seasoning and enjoy!

Risotto ai Gamberi (Shrimp Risotto)

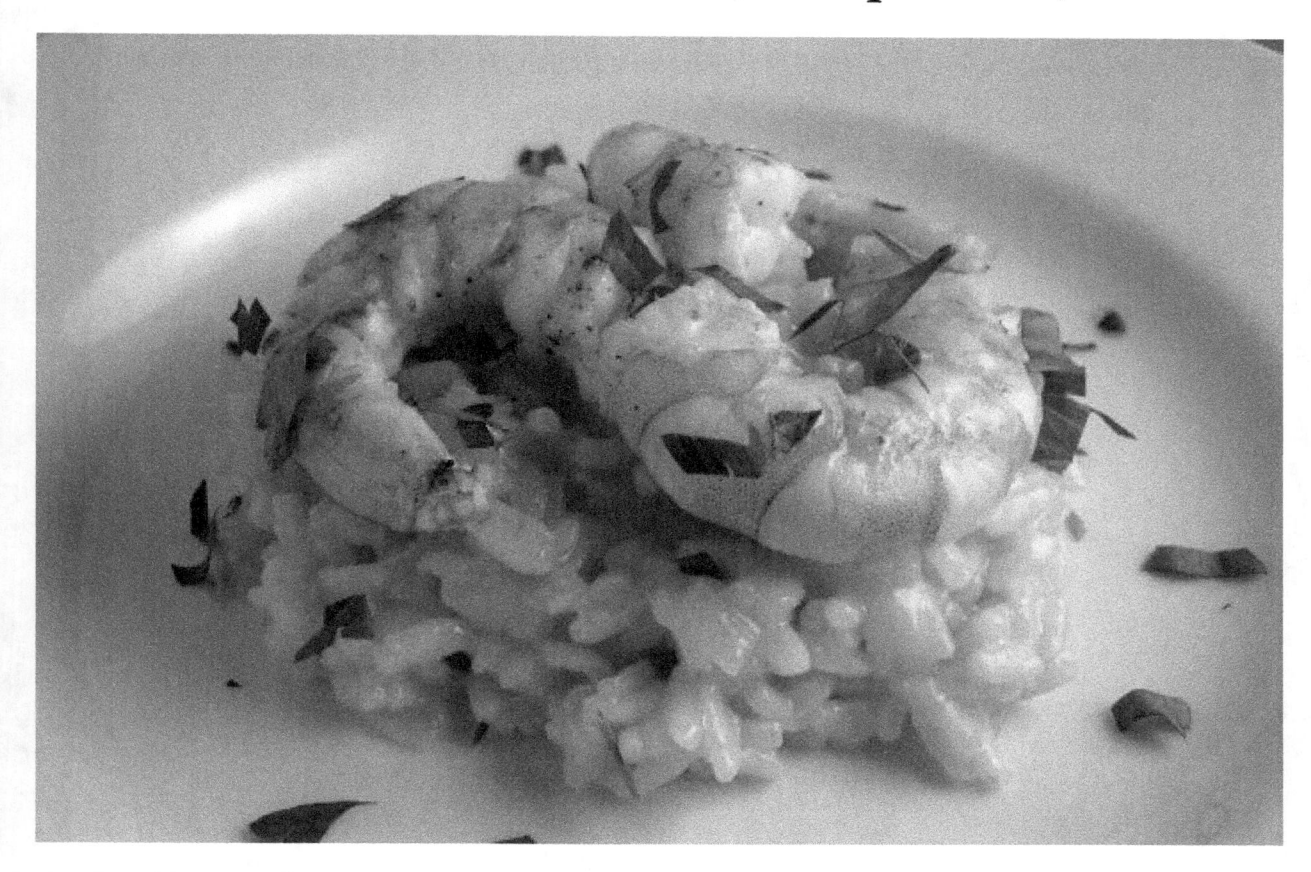

On the table you will see a steaming bowl of risotto covered in shrimp. Oh yes! This is something special. The rich color of tomato and onion sauce with an array of cooked shrimp laying on top really catches the eye and the hunger.

 I don't believe anyone could resist such a sight. Go for it. The messier the better.

<u>Total</u>: 60 minutes

<u>Prep Time</u>: 15 minutes

<u>Cooking Time</u>: 45 minutes

<u>Serving Size</u>: 6 servings

Ingredients	Measurements
Risotto rice	2 cups
Deveined medium to large full shrimp	1 lb
Dry white wine	¾ cup
Yellow onion	1 medium
Tomato paste	1 tbsp
Tomato puree	1 cup
Fresh parsley	2 sprigs + 1 cup
Red pepper flakes	pinch
Water	7 cups
Garlic	2 cloves
Lemon	1
Olive oil	¼ cup
Salt and pepper	pinch

Special Equipment:

- Dutch oven

Directions:

1. Begin by cleaning the shrimp and keeping your shrimp heads and shells for the broth you will be making.
2. Cut each shrimp into quarters and place them into a small bowl with salt to season. Refrigerate for later.
3. In your Dutch oven, heat 2 tbsp of olive oil on medium to high heat. Once simmering, add in your reserved shrimp shells and heads and cook for 5 minutes until the shells become a deep orange color.
4. Take your onion and halve it, dicing one half and finely chopping the other.
5. Introduce the diced onion and both crushed garlic cloves, stirring for 3 to 5 minutes until it browns.
6. Add in your tomato paste and fresh parsley sprigs. Cook for approximately 1 minute until the tomato starts to stick to the pot.
7. Add in only ¼ cup of the white wine while using a wooden spoon to scrape off the burnt bits. Add in all the water, bring it to a hard boil, and then lower heat to a simmer for 10 minutes.
8. Now take a fine-mesh strainer over a large bowl and strain the contents ensuring no liquids are wasted; set aside. Remove the shrimp shells and other solids.
9. Quickly give your Dutch oven a clean so that you may begin preparing your risotto rice.
10. Next, set the remaining 2 tbsp of olive oil on medium heat in your clean Dutch oven and add in the other half of your finely chopped onion. Season well with salt and pepper and stir for 5 minutes until the onion is glossy but not burnt.

11. Increase heat to medium-high and add in your rice and keep stirring until consistently coated for 2 to 3 minutes. Then add in your red pepper flakes and the remaining white wine and cook for 30 seconds until almost completely evaporated.
12. Now we can add in the tomato puree and half of the retained shrimp stock. Season with some salt and cook for 2 minutes until thickened slightly.
13. Keep adding the stock in 1/2 cup increments and slowly stir for 15 minutes.
14. Add in the cut shrimp and another ½ cup of stock. Reduce the heat to medium and cook for 2 minutes more. The rice should still be swimming in the stock.
15. Season with some more salt, add in the finely chopped parsley and serve immediately with quartered lemon wedges.

Nifty Tips:

- Always make sure your shrimp are thoroughly de-veined and de-shelled before use.

- If guests are not squeamish, reserve a couple of heads per portion for it to be plated. They are delicious and juicy!

Risotto With Walnuts and Blue Cheese

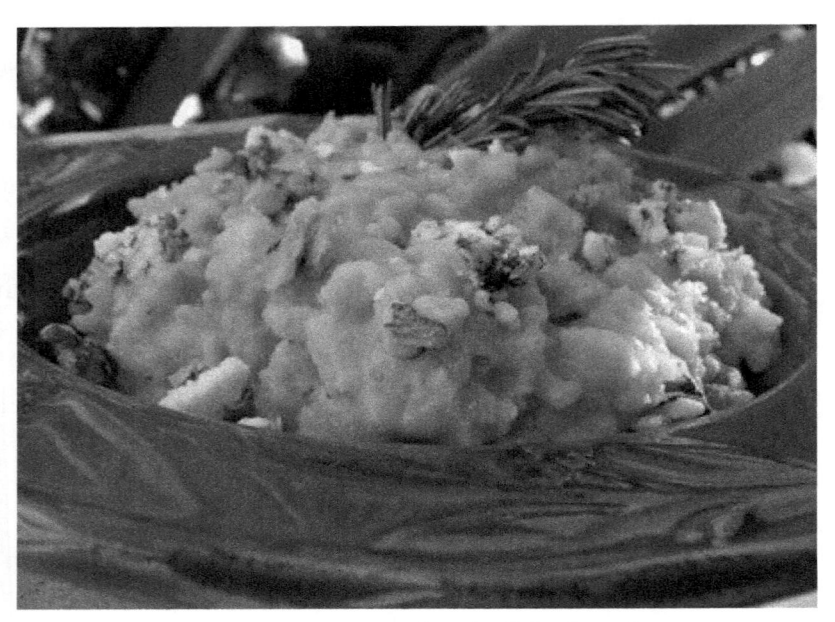

On the table you will see a steaming bowl of thick sticky risotto. You can already smell the fragrant aroma of walnuts and the beautifully pungent smell of gorgonzola. The two ingredients together bring about a dish that is wonderfully rich and warm. Then, you will taste the radicchio and its bitter twist to the combination. Wow!

Total: 40 minutes
Prep Time: 15 minutes
Cooking Time: 25 minutes
Serving Size: 4 servings

Ingredients	Measurements
Risotto rice	2 cups
Radicchio	7 oz (1 head)
Walnut halves	1 cup
Dry red or white wine	1 cup
Chicken or vegetable stock	4 cups
Parmesan cheese	2 oz (cups)
Gorgonzola cheese	garnish
Shallots	2 large 5 oz
Fresh thyme	1 tsp
Olive oil	5 tbsp
Salt and pepper	pinch

Directions:

1. Start by mixing the rice and the stock in a large bowl for around 1 minute. This will help release the starch from the rice. Strain well for 5 minutes, stirring the rice occasionally, and keep the stock aside.
2. Over medium-high heat, add in 3 tbsp of olive oil to a medium saucepan until it starts shimmering. Then add in your risotto rice and brown for 5 minutes.
3. Add in your minced shallots and carry on stirring for 1 minute. Then pour in your wine and cook for another 30 seconds until mostly evaporated.
4. Give the set aside stock a good stir and pour all but one cup over the rice. Increase heat to high and simmer. Then stir only once and cover with a lid to let it sit at the lowest setting for 10 minutes. Stir one more time, then cover again for a further 10 minutes.
5. In the meantime, in a small pan, heat the remaining olive oil over medium heat while adding the hand-crushed walnuts for 2 minutes until golden and aromatic.
6. Sprinkle in your chopped thyme and toss vigorously. Season with a pinch of salt and pepper and remove from the heat.
7. You will now want to remove the lid from the rice and add in the last cup of stock along with the washed and thinly sliced radicchio leaves. Increase your heat to high, stirring until it becomes thicker and creamier.
8. Remove from the heat, add salt and pepper, and add the grated parmesan to taste. Dish with the walnut mix, crumbly gorgonzola, and more grated parmesan if need be.

Nifty Tips:

- Avoid drying out the risotto when cooking by always keeping a minimal moisture level in the pot.

Chapter 11: Polenta and Frittata

In this chapter I would like to bring to your attention the beauty of yellow cornmeal. Polenta is a traditional beauty with a taste that is unique and maybe takes a little getting used to. If you have the right sauce and the right meat, you can make magic. Served as a porridge or as a solidified loaf, it sucks up any juices on your plate and can change your life in one bite.

What I will also be showing you is a quick couple of recipes for a frittata. Frittata is a type of omelet crossed with a quiche that is usually filled with a variety of fresh and creamy flavors. This fried egg quiche is wonderful warm or cold and can be eaten at any time of day.

Smooth and Creamy Polenta

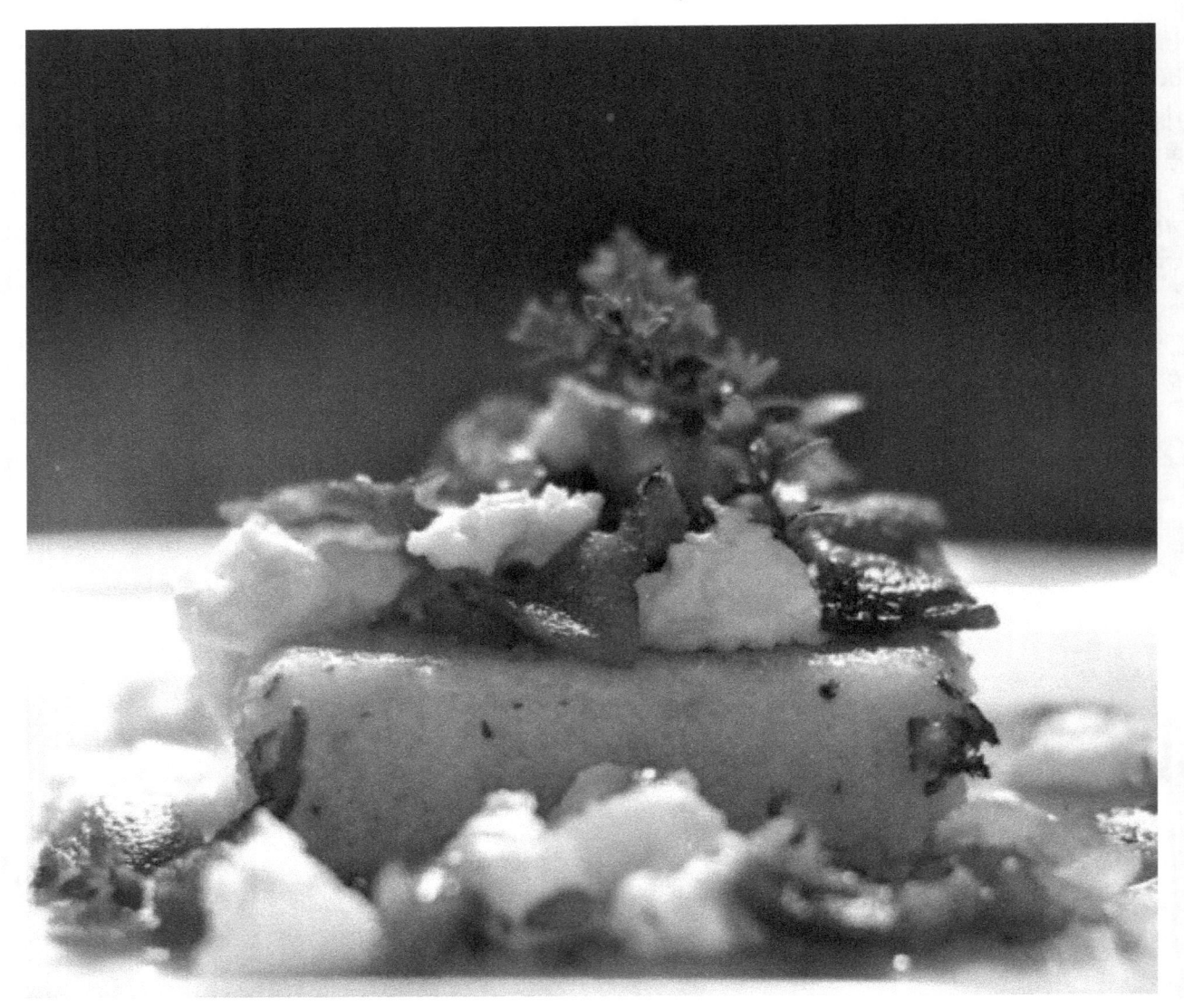

On the table you will see a bowl of what looks like yellow porridge. This dish could look incredibly foreign to someone who has never had it before, but when you take your first bite, you will be swept away by a creaminess and softness that cannot be compared to any other type of meal you have probably ever had.

This unique dish is a must-try for the curious and creative.

Total: 75 minutes
Prep Time: 15 minutes
Cooking Time: 60 minutes
Serving Size: 4 to 6 servings

Ingredients	Measurements
Medium or coarse polenta	1 cup
Chicken or vegetable stock	5 cups
Olive oil	2 tbsp
Salt and pepper	Pinch

<u>Directions</u>:

1. In a medium saucepan, warm up the stock over high heat.
2. Add in your polenta, stirring continuously, then bring to a hard boil.
3. When you start seeing the polenta split open, reduce the heat immediately so that it can thicken without further splitting.
4. As you keep stirring constantly, also make sure to scrape the bottom of the pan with a wooden spoon to prevent burning.
5. Polenta should thicken as it pulls away from the saucepan and congeals, which takes around 50 minutes. Sprinkle a little salt.
6. Pour in your olive oil and proceed to whisk the polenta till it creates a somewhat creamy, smooth, and glossy appearance. Serve with whatever sauce topping you like best.

<u>Nifty Tips</u>:

- You will know that the polenta is cooked when it starts cracking open.

- Add small amounts of water to the polenta if it's getting too thick.

- You can grill or sear this polenta base for more variation and texture in the recipe.

Polenta Concia

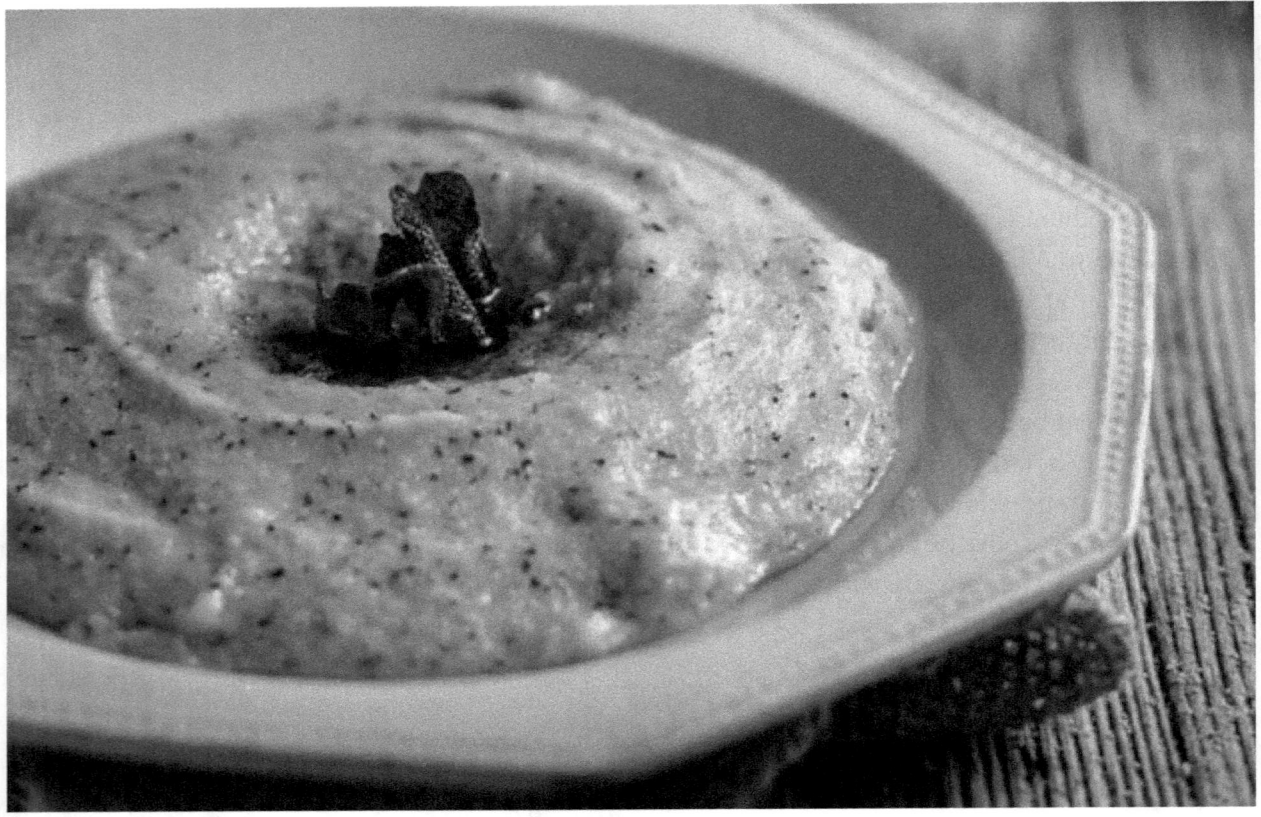

This Photo by Unknown Author is licensed under CC BY-NC-ND

On the table you will see a large dish of white creamy polenta. It is simple in itself, but as you smell the wonderful melted Fontina, you will become simply hooked. *Concia* means tan, so the name of this recipe tells us that it is a wonderfully tanned polenta.

This is another recipe that is simple in its foundation but needs a little more time cooking to really show its true colors.

Total: 50 minutes
Prep Time: 5 minutes
Cooking Time: 45 minutes
Serving Size: 4 to 6 servings

Ingredients	Measurements
Polenta	250g (1 cup)
Water	4 cups
Whole milk	¾ cup
Fontina	1 cup
Unsalted butter	1 cup
Salt and pepper	pinch

Directions:

1. Firstly, bring your large pot of heavily salted water to a boil and mix in the polenta, cooking for 45 minutes. Keep stirring to remove lumps.
2. Take your Fontina cheese, make sure to de-rind, and then cut into small cubes.
3. Now you will slowly add your milk to the polenta pot and keep stirring to thin out the consistency. Then add in the butter and cheese, turning until melted.
4. Season with salt and pepper and serve.

Nifty Tips:

- Add a little more water to the polenta to create the desired consistency.

Classic Italian Frittata

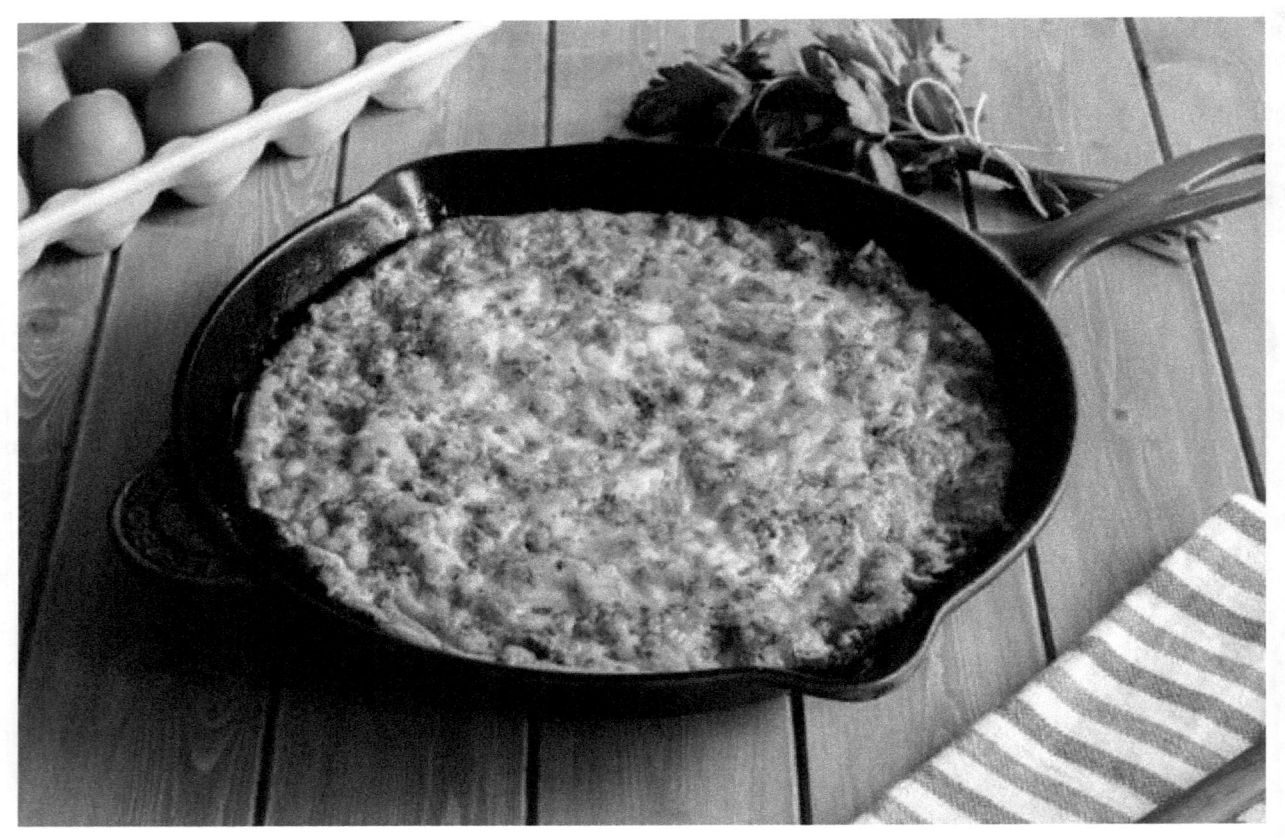

On the table you will see a large dish with an oversized and rounded omelet. Yes, that is definitely egg, and what is that inside? Well, you will just have to bite in to find out.

The gorgeous saltiness of salami hits you first, then the texture of the artichoke and the earthiness of the mushrooms. Now you can taste all those cheeses imbued in the cooked egg and the slight garlic and onion vigor as well. What a beauty!

<u>Total</u>: 50 minutes

<u>Prep Time</u>: 25 minutes

<u>Cooking Time</u>: 25 minutes

<u>Serving Size</u>: 6 servings

Ingredients	Measurements
Eggs	6
Artichoke hearts	½ cup
Italian salami	½ cup
Mushrooms	4 ½ oz
Green onions	2
Onion powder	1 tsp
Cherry tomatoes	½ cup
Mozzarella cheese	1 cup
Parmesan cheese	⅓ cup
Whole milk	⅓ cup
Garlic	1 clove
Dried basil	1 tsp
Olive oil	1 tsp
Salt and pepper	Pinch

Directions:

1. We shall start by preheating the oven to 425 °F (220 °C).
2. Then take a medium baking dish and grease with some butter or spray and cook.
3. Then take a pan over medium heat, add in your olive oil, and drop in your diced salami, your drained and chopped artichoke hearts, your chopped cherry tomatoes, and your sliced mushrooms. Saute for 4 minutes and then move the mix into your greased baking dish.
4. In a separate bowl, whisk the eggs, chopped onions, minced garlic, and milk. Sprinkle in your onion powder, dried basil, and salt and pepper.
5. Pour the whisked egg mixture over the salami in the baking dish and sprinkle on top grated mozzarella and parmesan.
6. Pop it into the oven for 20 minutes until the cheese is bubbling and eggs are fully cooked.

Nifty Tips:

- Use any kind of mushroom you prefer. You can choose canned, but it is ideal if fresh.

Potato Frittata

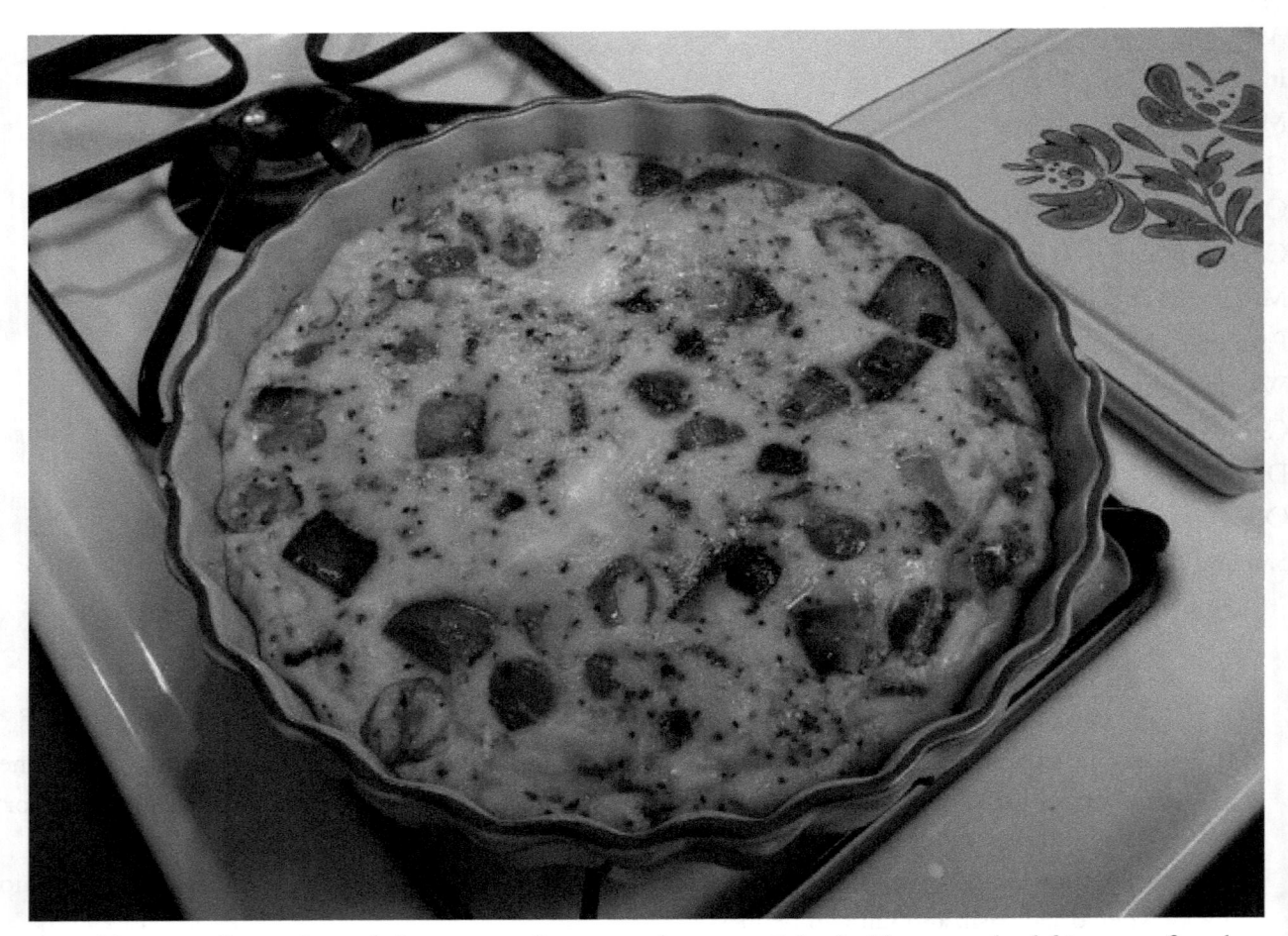

On the table you will see a large dish serving a frittata with a twist. It looks like a standard frittata at first, but as you cut into it, you can see chunky pieces of potato within the cooked egg.

This is simple, but potatoes elevate the whole dish at once. A must-try!

Total: 30 minutes
Prep Time: 10 minutes
Cooking Time: 20 minutes
Serving Size: 6 servings

Ingredients	Measurements
Eggs	6
Potatoes	500g (2 cups)
Fresh parsley	handful
Olive oil	3 tbsp
Parmesan cheese	½ cups
Salt and pepper	pinch

<u>Directions</u>:

1. Begin by peeling and chopping the potatoes into 1 inch cubes.
2. Bring a large pot of salted water to a boil, add in your potatoes, and cook for 5 minutes. Drain the potatoes and set aside.
3. Now in a large bowl, whisk your eggs well, sprinkle in your chopped parsley, add in salt and pepper and stir.
4. Take your drained potatoes and pop them into the bowl with your egg mix, then gently fold in the grated cheese and mix well.
5. Take your skillet and heat to low to medium heat, with a touch of olive oil. Pour in the frittata mixture, making sure the potatoes are evenly dispersed in the skillet.
6. Cover and cook for 10 minutes. Every now and then, shake the skillet to release the egg. When you can easily lift the egg off the pan, you know it is ready to be turned to cook the other side.
7. Cook uncovered for 10 minutes and then place it on a serving plate. Slice accordingly and serve.

<u>Nifty Tips</u>:

- A great technique to turn your frittata is to place a plate over the skillet and support the frittata with the plate while you turn it. This removes the chance of an ugly mess.

Chapter 12: Pizza and Other Doughs

If I had a quarter for every time someone told me that pizza was their favorite food, well, let's say I'd be a little richer for sure!

Who doesn't love the crispy pizza crust, the rich yet subtle tomato base, and the countless ingredients that you can choose from to top it all off? It is an incredibly versatile food that pleases almost any palate, so why go order one when you can make it at home with love?

In this chapter, we will go through a couple of simple pizza recipes, but what we will also do is touch on one of my favorite flatbread recipes and a stunning calzone dish that will truly blow your friends away.

Classic Margherita Pizza

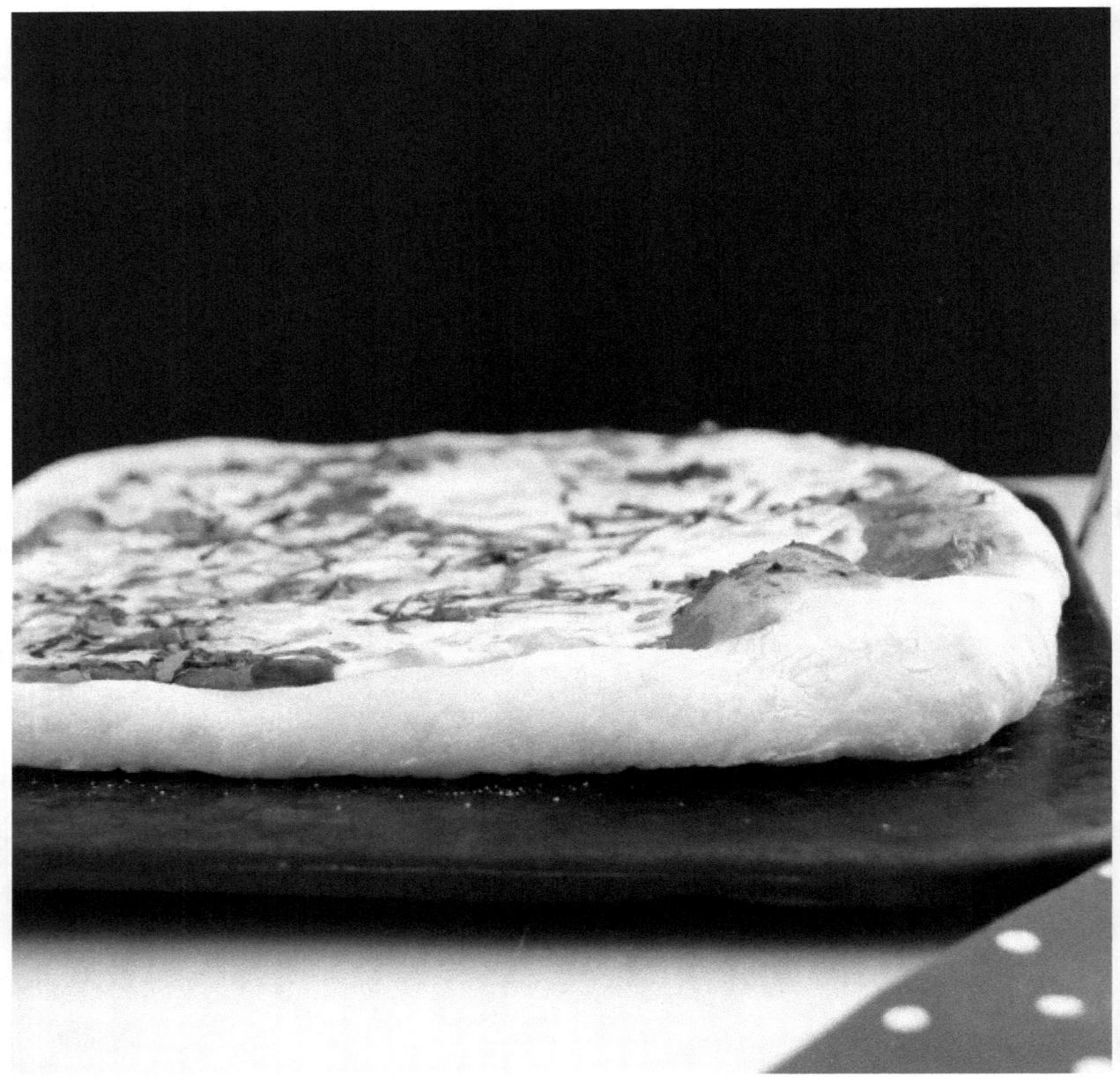

This Photo by Unknown Author is licensed under CC BY

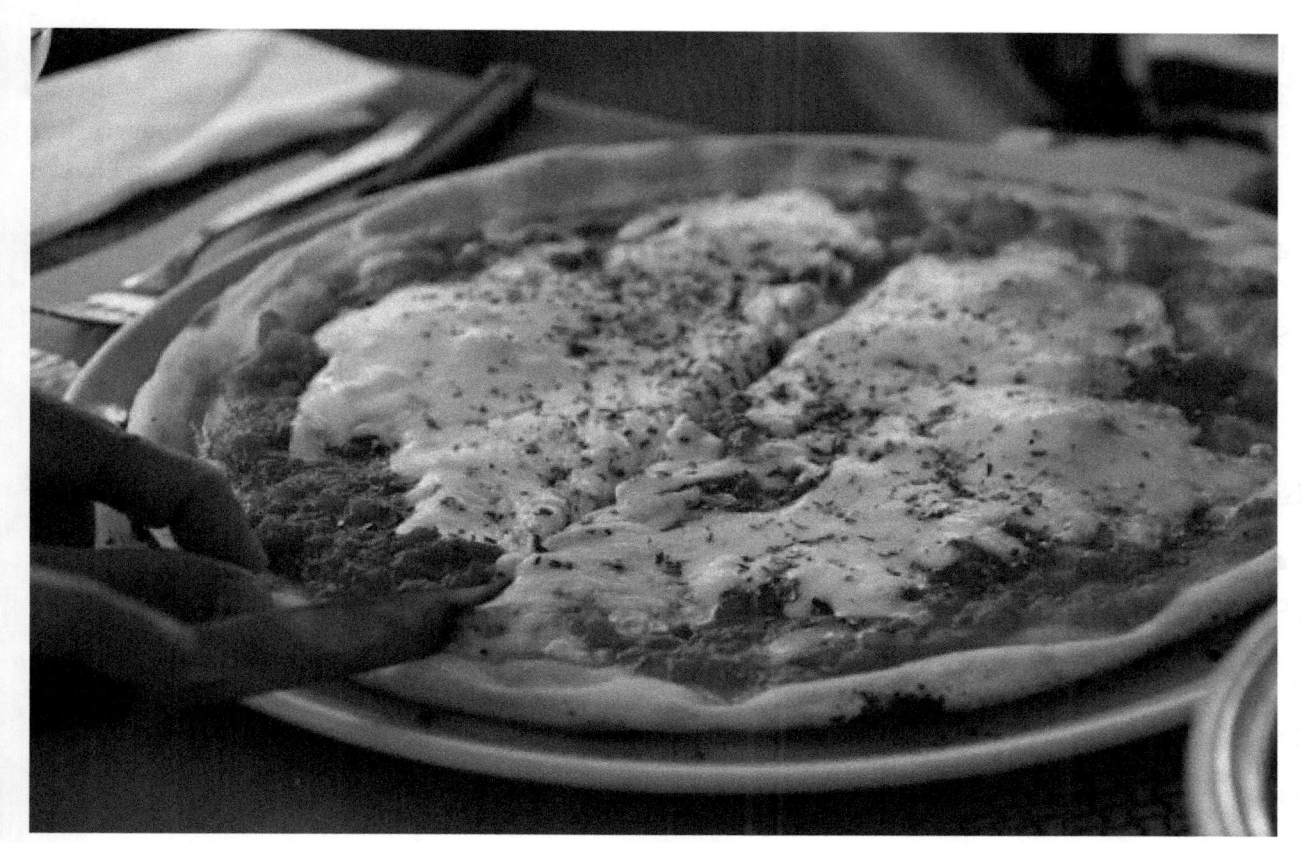

On the table you will see a pizza that you can certainly recognize with ease. The classic and everlasting Margherita pizza has become the poster child to most Italian restaurant logos and is a great recipe to make at home.

Total: 25 minutes

Prep Time: 10 minutes (includes resting)

Cooking Time: 20 minutes

Serving Size: 4 servings

Ingredients	Measurements
Pizza dough	1 (base)
Mozzarella	4 oz
Crushed tomatoes	12 oz (1 can)
Cherry tomatoes	5
Fresh basil leaves	10 leaves
Salt and pepper	Pinch

Special Equipment:

- Pizza stone (ceramic baking stone)
- Pizza cutter

Directions:

1. Begin by cutting a length out of your baking paper in the size of your pizza stone and set it aside.
2. Preheat your oven to 500 °F (260 °C) and place your pizza stone within.
3. Lightly flour your baking paper and place the premade pizza base on top. Evenly pour out your crushed tomato over the base, spreading with the back of a spoon in a circular motion from the center to the rim of the base.
4. Grab your pizza cutter and slice through the dough at the desired proportions. Pop in the oven on top of the pizza stone for 15 minutes until the crust starts to thoroughly crisp.
5. Now you can top with the grated mozzarella cheese and cook for a further 5 minutes. Allow the pizza to sit for another 5 minutes to bring about a sticky cheese texture and then add on your chopped cherry tomatoes and roughly torn basil before you serve.

Nifty Tips:

- When adding in your fresh garnish of any kind, you will want to tear rather than cut to increase the flavor surface area.

Sausage and Arugula Pizza

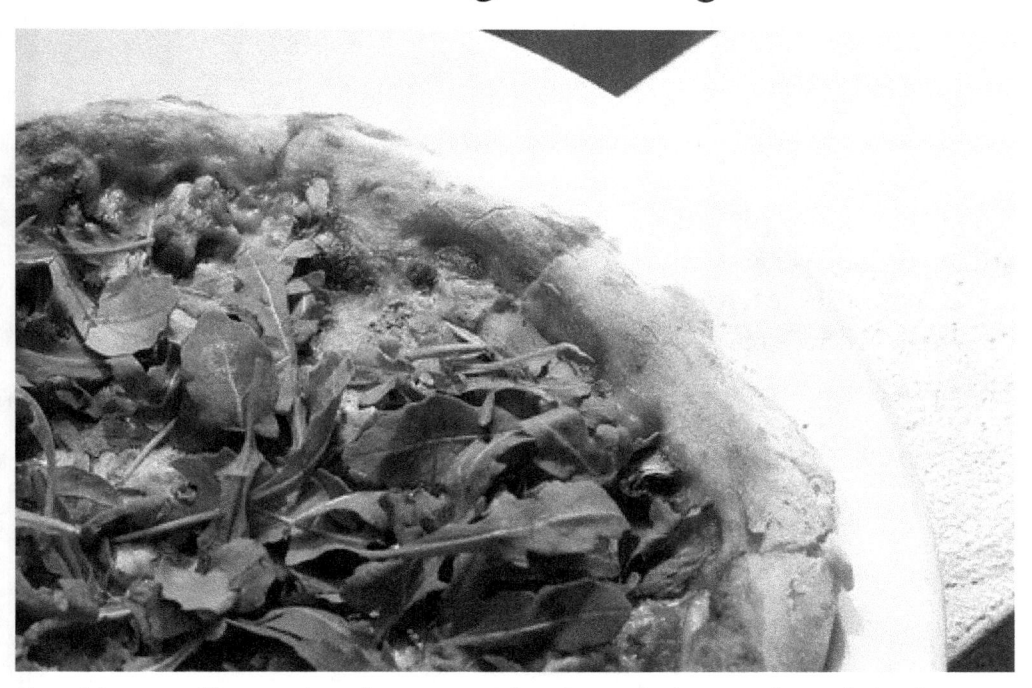

On the table you will see a pizza that pops with color and vibrancy. Arugula is what some like to call rocket, and its bitter taste truly brings something special out of a rich and saucy base, especially with the topped sausage.

Total: 32 minutes

Prep Time: 20 minutes

Cooking Time: 12 minutes

Serving Size: 4 servings

Ingredients	Measurements
Pizza dough	1 base
Mozzarella	½ cup
Fresh arugula	1 cup
Unsalted tomato sauce	¼ cup
Pork sausage	4 oz
Dried thyme	½ tsp
Garlic powder	2 tsp
Olive oil	2 tbsp
Salt and pepper	Pinch

Special Equipment:

- Pizza stone

Directions:

1. Before you begin, make sure to cook your sausage through and remove the casing before adding to the recipe.
2. Then preheat the oven to 450° F (230 °C) with the pizza stone inside.
3. Cut a length out of your baking paper in the size of your pizza stone and put it aside.
4. Lightly flour your baking paper and place the premade pizza base on top. Evenly pour your unsalted tomato sauce on top, spreading evenly with the back of a spoon.
5. Sprinkle your dried thyme and garlic powder, then add your grated mozzarella cheese.
6. Add your cooked sausage and bake for around 12 minutes until the crust starts to puff up and char.
7. Remove from the oven and drizzle olive oil while popping on the lightly chopped fresh arugula leaves; serve immediately.

Nifty Tips:

- You can use a pizza stone or you can use a baking tray.

Zucchini and Herbed Ricotta Flatbread

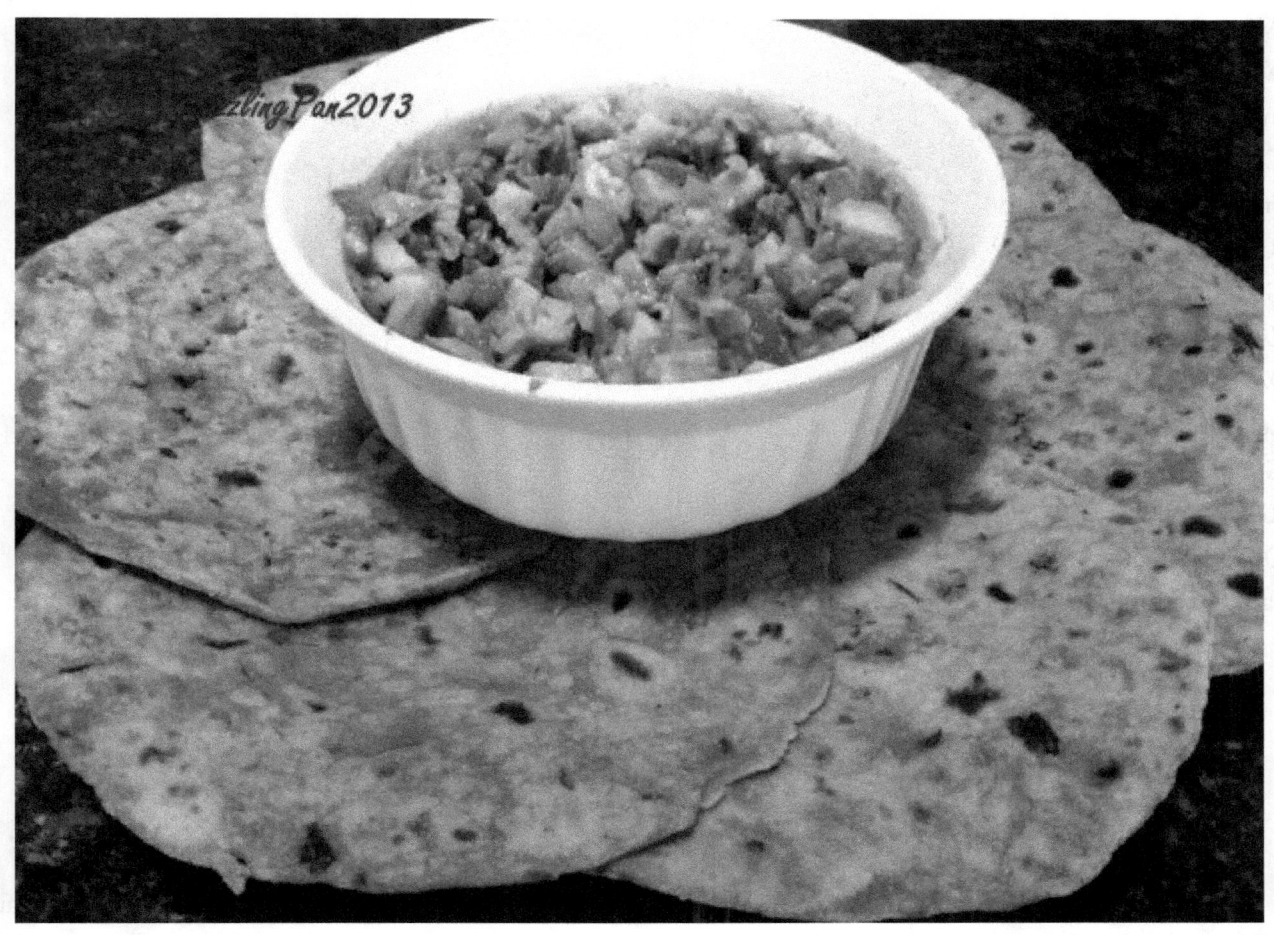

On the table you will see a flatbread that holds so much flavor, it is surprising. The visual aspect of the dish is amazing as is, but when you bite in you receive the creaminess of the herbed ricotta and goat cheese, along with the unmistakable flavor of fresh zucchini.

This is a wonderful vegetarian pizza for the family to enjoy together.

Total: 1 hour 20 minutes

Prep Time: 1 hour

Cooking Time: 20 minutes

Serving Size: 4 servings

Ingredients	Measurements
AP flour	2 cups
Warm water	¾ cup
White sugar	1 tsp
Instant yeast	1 tsp
Cherry tomatoes	1 cups
Fresh basil	3 tbsp
Ricotta cheese	2 cups
Goat cheese	6 to 8 oz
Zucchini	2 cups
Whole milk	2 tbsp
Lemon juice	2 tbsp
Garlic	2 tsp
Red pepper flakes	pinch
Olive oil	4 tbsp
Salt and pepper	pinch

Special Equipment:

- Food processor with dough paddle
- Pizza stone

Directions:

1. Preheat your oven to 400 °F (204 °C) with the pizza stone inside. Cut a length out of your baking paper the size of your pizza stone and put it aside.
2. Begin by making the flatbread by adding in your food processor the flour, 1 tbsp of olive oil, and a pinch of salt. At the lowest speed, mix for 1 minute till well combined in a rough dough ball.
3. On a lightly floured surface, knead the dough for around 2 minutes till slightly smooth. Then place the dough in a medium greased bowl, covered, to rise for 45 minutes.
4. In the meanwhile, we can begin preparing the toppings by grabbing a medium bowl and adding in your halved cherry tomatoes along with 1 tbsp of olive oil. Sprinkle salt and pepper and toss.
5. On a lined baking tray, place your tomatoes and bake for 20 minutes until they are soft and charred, then set aside. Turn the oven heat up to 475 °F (246 °C).
6. Now take a medium bowl and add in the crumbled ricotta, chopped basil, lemon juice, milk, and minced garlic. Whisk thoroughly and set aside.
7. It's time to take your risen dough and place it on a floured surface. Compress the dough to release excess air bubbles and divide it into 2 sections.
8. Each section should be pulled and stretched into a ¼ inch thickness. Then transfer the bases to the pre-

cut baking paper and use your fingers to create dimples in the dough. Brush with ½ tsp olive oil.
9. Add your ricotta mixture on each base and top with your fresh sliced zucchini, charred tomatoes, and crumbled goat cheese. Return to the oven for 15 minutes to crisp. Slice and serve.

<u>Nifty Tips</u>:

- You can use a skim or full-fat ricotta cheese. The difference will be in the thickness and richness of the course.

- Don't stress too much about the shape being perfect. The beauty of a flatbread is its crispy and uneven visual appeal.

- You can use a knife to poke the base instead of your fingers.

Calzone With Ricotta and Prosciutto

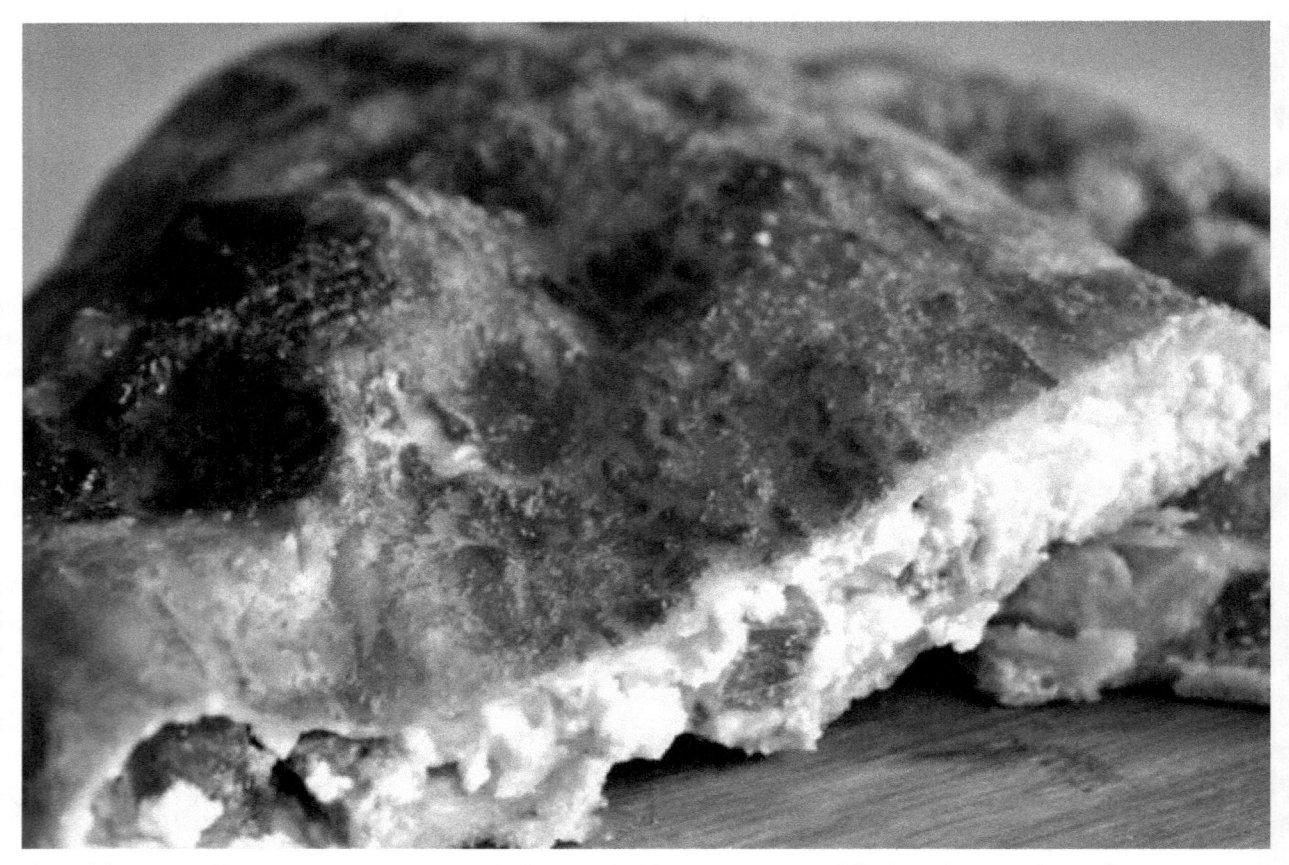

On the table you will see a very interesting dish. This half-moon pizza is filled with something divine. The smell is incredible and you will not be able to wait to cut it open. And yes, that is prosciutto, with its distinct saltiness, then soft ricotta combined with the stronger and flavorsome pecorino cheese. Tomatoes and olives too!

Basically, this is a pizza that has been closed shut!

Total: 3 hours 25 minutes

Prep Time: 3 hours (includes rising)

Baking Time: 25 minutes

Serving Size: 1 to 2 servings

Ingredients	Measurements
00 flour	5 cups
Active yeast	1 ½ tbsp
Room temperature water	400 ml
Whole tomatoes	1 cup
Fresh ricotta	½ cup
Mozzarella	½ lb
Prosciutto	⅓ lb
Pecorino	¼ cup
Olive oil	1 tbsp
Salt	2 tbsp
Salt and pepper	pinch

<u>Special Equipment</u>:

- Food processor
- Pizza stone

<u>Directions</u>:

1. Begin by making the calzone dough. In your food processor, add in the water and 1 ½ tbsp of salt. Mix for around 1 minute on high, then crumble in your active yeast and mix for another 90 seconds.
2. Change the speed setting to medium and add in your flour one cup at a time, slowly watching as it mixes consistently. Then let it mix fully for another 12 minutes.
3. Grab your medium bowl, lightly flour it, and place in your dough ball, covering with plastic wrap. Let it rise for 45 minutes at room temperature.
4. Once the dough has made its first rise, you can separate the dough ball in half, re-form each into its own ball, and place each in a separate covered bowl to rise and proof for another 45 minutes.
5. Around 10 minutes before the last proof is complete, turn on your oven and preheat it to 400 °F (205 °C). Now take your baking paper and grease it with some olive oil; set it aside.
6. On a floured surface, begin to knead each ball into a flattened round about ½ inch thick. It should be large enough to hold your ingredients and be folded in two.
7. On each base, and centered as much as possible, place your chopped mozzarella, ⅓ cup of grated pecorino, thinly sliced prosciutto slices, and fresh ricotta. Sprinkle a little salt and pepper and proceed to fold each segment in half, pinching the edges closed with wet fingers. This should create 2 half-moon parcels ready to bake. Place each on the baking paper.
8. Before you bake, coat the calzone with the crushed tomatoes, sprinkle the remaining pecorino, drizzle some olive oil, and add a pinch of salt and pepper. Place both calzones on the hot pizza stone in the oven for 25 minutes. Once done, serve immediately.

Nifty Tips:

- You can use instant yeast as well. That would mean you do not have to insert it into the water mix but rather straight into the flour mix.

- Using 00 flour will give the calzone its typical robust texture and distinct flavor, although, using AP flour will not ruin the recipe.

Chapter 13: Seafood, Poultry, and Meats

Why do seafood, chicken, and beef have such a distinct variation in Italian cuisine? Why are they usually accompanied as pasta or a soup, and why do they differ from the typical protein meals we see all around the world?

I will be bringing to you an array of classic dishes that represent Italian cuisine in terms of all three proteins. When you see how these are prepared, and in what portion, you will have a better idea of how Italians like eating their protein and why.

Let's take a look at some of the more common seafood, chicken, and beef dishes.

Salt-Baked Whole Fish With Fresh Herbs

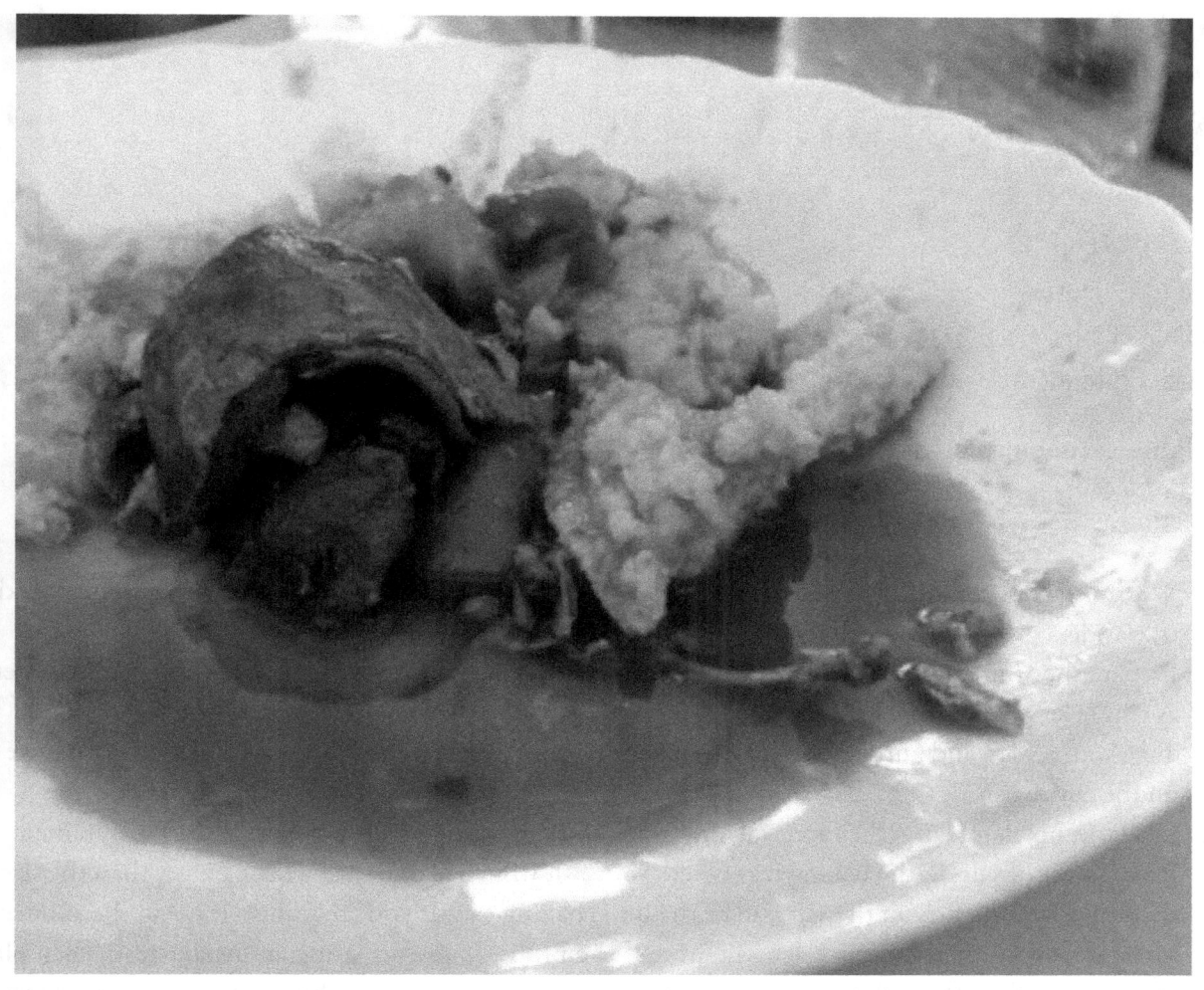

On the table you will see a fish that has been cooked to perfection. There is a fragrant aroma that accompanies the sweet fish that invites you in. This fish is cooked in a very specific way for it to be so juicy and so flavorful.

Total: 40 minutes

Prep Time: 10 minutes

Cooking Time: 30 minutes

Serving Size: 2 to 4 servings

Ingredients	Measurements
Whole fish	2 lb
Kosher salt	2 lb
Fresh parsley	Handful
Fresh ginger	Handful
Fresh thyme	Handful
Lemon	½
Water	¾ cup
Garlic	2 cloves
Olive oil	1 tsp

Special Equipment:

- Probe thermometer (leave-in or instant-read)

Directions:

1. We can start by preheating the oven to a good 400 °F (205 °C) and setting a lined and rimmed baking tray aside.
2. Prepare the aromatic stuffing by peeling the garlic cloves and slicing the ginger, keeping the fresh herbs as whole leaves and sprigs.
3. Take your scaled and gutted fish and begin stuffing your aromatics into the cavity. Then brush olive oil on the entire fish.
4. In a large bowl, mix together your salt and water until a malleable but not wet mixture is obtained.
5. Pack a layer of salt on the baking tray where your fish will be placed, just a little bigger than the size of the fish. Place the fish on the salt bed of the lined baking tray. If you are using a leave-in thermometer, insert it now so that you can pack salt around the probe. If you are using an instant-read, then place the probe in the fish, pack the salt around it, and gently remove the probe so a hole is created for later temperature checks.
6. Once you have tightly packed your fish with the remaining salt, place it in the oven to bake for 30 minutes. Keep checking the temperature and make sure to remove the fish when it reaches 130 °F (55 °C). Let it rest for 5 minutes.
7. Using a sharp knife, cut open the salt at the belly. When cracking open the salt, the skin and the salt will peel away together. Therefore, make sure to not let the salt touch the white flesh when cleaning. Discard the salt and skin.
8. Now you can filet the fish and serve with a couple of lemon wedges.

Nifty Tips:

- Choose a fish such as bass, dorde, snapper, branzino, or trout.

- Keep in mind that when you bake a fish in a salt crust, the fish can easily overcook in the enclosure's salt seal. Thanks to the food probe, you can keep an eye on the internal temperature of the fish.

- Do not overstuff with aromatics, as this could overpower the flavor of the fish.

- Using a leave-in probe is a better way to work with time as you can just check the reading without having to open the oven throughout the bake.

- You can use either water or egg whites to moisten the salt. Both work great.

Osso Buco

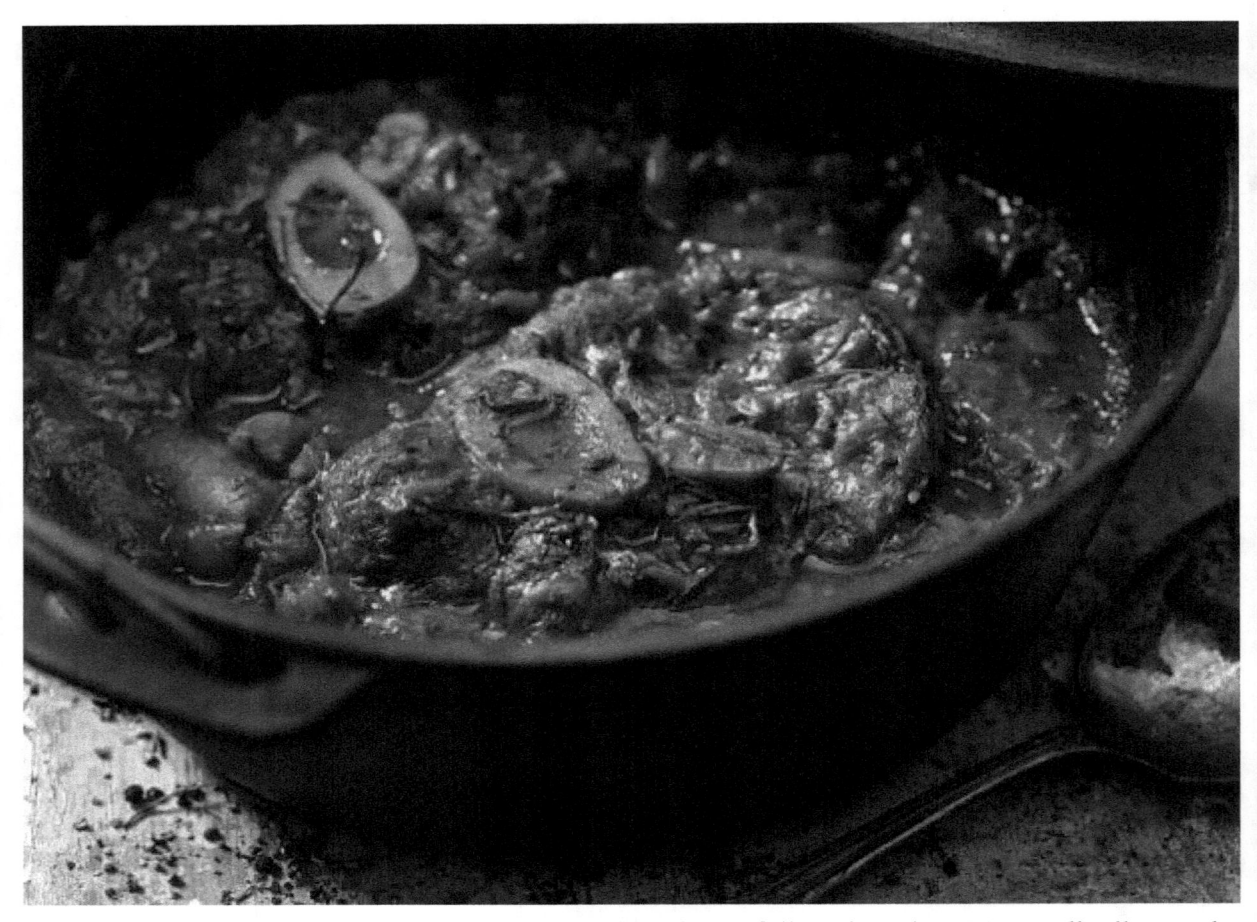

On the table, you will see a large dish that has something beautifully rich within. The smell tells you that it is meat, and by the looks of it, that meat is as tender and juicy as they come. Swimming in a thick tomato and herb sauce, you cannot help but grab a spoon and begin plating for yourself.

Veal shanks in a base like this are something you won't just cook once.

Total: 4 hours

Prep Time: 45 minutes

Cooking Time: 3 hours 15 minutes

Serving Size: 6 servings

Ingredients	Measurements
Veal shanks	6 (4 lb)
Peeled whole tomatoes	1 can (28 oz)
Dry white wine	1 cup
AP flour	1 cup
Carrots	2 medium
Yellow onion	1
Celery	1 rib
Fresh thyme	3 sprigs
Fresh parsley	2 tbsp
Bay leaf	1
Garlic	9 cloves
Chicken stock	¾ cup
Unsalted butter	½ oz
Lemon	1
Olive oil	¼ cup
Salt and pepper	big pinch

Special Equipment:

- Dutch oven

Directions:

1. Begin by preheating your oven to 325 °F (163 °C).
2. Season the shanks with a light coating of salt and pepper and set them aside.
3. Grab a shallow bowl, add in your flour, and set aside.
4. Heat your Dutch oven at medium-high temperature and add in your olive oil. Now coat your shanks lightly in flour, making sure to shake off any excess from the surface. Add these to the heated oil in batches.
5. Turn the shanks every now and then until all are brown on both sides, adding some oil as you go. This should be around 4 minutes. Once all batches are cooked, set aside on a plate.
6. Return to your Dutch oven, heat up the butter, and insert the finely chopped onion, carrots, celery, and 3 of your minced garlic cloves. Saute for 6 minutes until lightly golden.
7. Now add in your hand crushed tomatoes, chicken stock, and wine. Drop in your veal shanks and their sitting juices, making sure shanks are spread out evenly.
8. Sprinkle in your thyme sprigs and bay leaf and allow this to reach a simmer. Prepare the parchment paper lid, place it over the shanks in the Dutch oven, make sure it covers the whole surface, tuck it into the edges, and bake for 2 hours.

9. While it bakes, prepare the gremolata sauce to go with the shanks. In a medium bowl, pop in the zest of 1 lemon, the remaining 6 minced garlic cloves, and the finely chopped parsley. Mix well and keep aside.
10. Remove the parchment lid from the Dutch oven, and place it back into the oven for another 1 hour. Check with a fork or knife to see if the meat is falling off the bone; make sure it is not completely dried out by adding in a little more stock while shifting the shanks around to expose them to more heat.
11. Around 20 minutes before the bake is done, stir in around 2 tsp of gremolata with the shanks, tasting as you go to your desired palate.
12. When completely cooked, remove the thyme and bay leaf, add a touch of stock if a little dry, and then serve with the remaining gremolata as a garnish. It helps to keep spoons at the table so the sauce can be enjoyed.

Nifty Tips:

- Make sure the butcher gets your veal cut between 1 to 1 ½ inch thick.

- If you want more compact and juicy meat, I highly recommend you tie each shank with butcher's string while it bakes.

- The accumulated juices should almost cover the shanks.

- To prepare a parchment paper lid, you will need to measure the size of your Dutch oven by cutting the parchment square accordingly. Fold the paper twice into a square, then roll it into a cone and cut off the tip. This should create a rounded shape with a hole in the center, almost like a coffee filter. The point of this exercise is to prevent the meat from reabsorbing any moisture as it cooks, allowing it to brown.

Slow Cooker Chicken Cacciatore

On the table you will see a large dish with juicy and creamy chicken pieces floating within. As you spoon some into your own bowl, you will see all the other ingredients that accompany the chicken. Peppers, mushrooms, and capers all play a large role in this marvelous dish.

The slow cooker this meal is cooked in will basically do all the chewing for you as the meat will fall off the bone and the sauce integrates perfectly with the chicken.

<u>Total</u>: 6 hours 10 minutes
<u>Prep Time</u>: 10 minutes
<u>Cooking Time</u>: 6 hours
<u>Serving Size</u>: 6 servings

Ingredients	Measurements
Chicken thighs with skin & bone	2 lb
Linguini pasta	8 oz
Chicken broth	½ cup
Bell peppers	2
Capers	⅓ cup
Baby Bella mushrooms	8 oz
Crushed tomatoes	28 oz (1 can)
Red pepper flakes	¼ tsp
Dried oregano	1 tsp
Garlic	2
Salt and pepper	pinch

<u>Special Equipment</u>:

- Slow cooker

<u>Directions</u>:

1. In your slow cooker at low heat, drop in your seasoned chicken thighs, chopped bell pepper, sliced mushrooms, minced garlic, and crushed tomatoes. Sprinkle in the oregano and the red pepper flakes and pour in your chicken stock. Sprinkle a little salt and pepper for taste and cook for 6 hours.
2. Around 20 minutes before the chicken is completely cooked, boil a medium pot of saltwater and cook your linguini till al dente. Drain and plate.
3. Remove the chicken from the slow cooker and place it on top of your plated pasta.
4. Grab your drained capers and stir them into the sauce for around 1 minute. Then spoon out your sauce onto the pasta and chicken. Garnish as desired and serve hot!

Nifty Tips:

- Remove your chicken skin if desired before it is placed into the slow cooker to decrease the greasiness.

Fritto Misto di Mare (Mix Fried Seafood Platter)

On the table you will see a dish that tells you good times are about to be had. An array of fried seafood awaits you, just reach out and grab what peaks your fancy first.

Hey, anything deep fried is on my menu! Tuck in.

<u>Total</u>: 45 minutes

<u>Prep Time</u>: 20 minutes

<u>Cooking Time</u>: 25 minutes

<u>Serving Size</u>: 6 serv

Ingredients	Measurements
Medium-large head-on shrimp	12 oz
Clean squid	1 lb
Clean smelt fish	12 oz
Semolina flour	2 cups
Sunflower oil	8 cups
Corn starch	½ cup
Lemon	2
Baking powder	½ tsp
Salt and pepper	pinch

<u>Special Equipment</u>:

- Dutch oven
- Spider skimmer spoon (used in frying)
- 2 wire racks with rimmed baking trays

<u>Directions</u>:

1. Let us begin by cleaning and deveining the shrimp, keeping the shells intact.
2. Now preheat the oven to 200 °F (95 °C).
3. Then grab your 2 baking trays, placing each wire rack inside. On one rack, place a calendar, and line the other rack with paper towel.
4. In your Dutch oven, heat your sunflower oil to 375 °F (190 °C).
5. While it heats up, grab a large bowl and whisk your flour, baking powder, and cornstarch together until well combined.
6. Take your squid tubes, clean, and pat dry with a paper towel. Cut each tube crosswise and keep your tentacles.
7. Toss your squid pieces into the flour mix and shake well so it coats completely. Place the squid into a colander and shake off the excess flour. Rest the floured squid on the paper towel wire rack.

8. Repeat this process with the cleaned smelt fish and the shrimp. Set aside.
9. Now we can begin deep-frying the seafood in batches by popping them into the Dutch oven oil for 2 to 3 minutes until golden brown. Remove the seafood with your spider skimmer and place it on paper towels to drain. Repeat the process with other seafood.
10. Serve on a large platter along with your lemons cut into wedges and sprinkled with salt and pepper.

<u>Nifty Tips</u>:

- If you are using frozen seafood, make sure it is completely defrosted and dried before frying.

- You can also use other small species like herring, capelin, or candlefish instead of smelt.

Tuscan Flank Steak

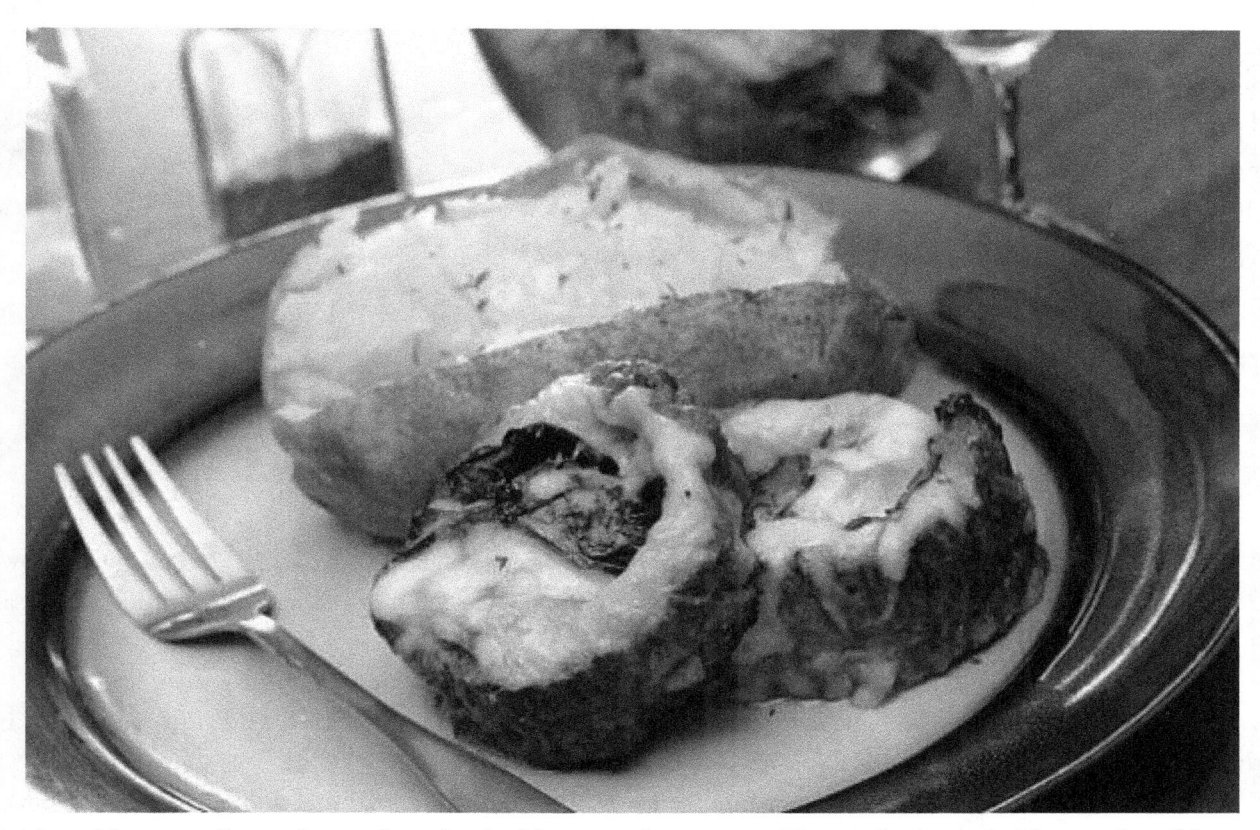

On the table you will see a large plate that holds a mouth-watering Tuscan flank steak. This steak will be so terribly juicy and aromatic that it would be hard to say no.

The flavor is without comparison because you have let this steak marinate overnight, bringing tenderness to the meat that you couldn't achieve without that patient wait.

<u>Total</u>: 4 hours 40 minutes
<u>Prep Time</u>: 20 minutes
<u>Cooking Time</u>: 14 minutes
<u>Serving Size</u>: 4 servings

Ingredients	Measurements
Trimmed flank steak	1 ½ lb
Fresh rosemary	½ cup + 1 tbsp
Fresh rosemary	1 sprig
Red pepper flakes	½ tsp
Lemon	1
Garlic	6 cloves
Olive oil	⅔ cup
Salt and pepper	big pinch

Special Equipment:

- Food processor

Directions:

1. In your food processor at medium speed, add in your ½ cup of chopped rosemary, whole garlic cloves, ⅓ cup olive oil, ¼ cup lemon juice, ¼ tsp red pepper flakes, a pinch of black pepper, and ½ tsp of salt. Blitz well until a smooth marinade appears, then set aside.
2. Take your steak and poke it with a fork around 20 times, place it in a baking dish, and pour the marinade over the steak. Turn the steak to thoroughly coat both sides. Then place the covered baking dish in the fridge between 4 to 8 hours.
3. Now to create the serving sauce, in a medium bowl, combine the remaining red pepper flakes, another ¼ cup of lemon juice, 1 tsp of minced rosemary, the remaining ⅓ cup of olive oil, zest from half the lemon, and a pinch of salt. Shake the bowl to combine the dressing, remembering to shake again just before use. Set aside.
4. Next, preheat your oven to grill setting, remove your steak from the marinade, make sure to take off any marinade chunks, and season with some salt and pepper. Discard the remaining marinade.
5. Place your steak in the oven for 6 to 8 minutes per side until nicely browned.
6. Once cooked, take your rosemary sprig and use it as a brush to baste your steak with the lemon and olive oil dressing. Let the steak sit for 5 minutes before slicing then drizzle with some olive oil and serve hot.

Nifty Tips:

- If you are using a meat thermometer you want the steak to show a temperature of 125°F (52 °C).

Classic Italian Meatballs

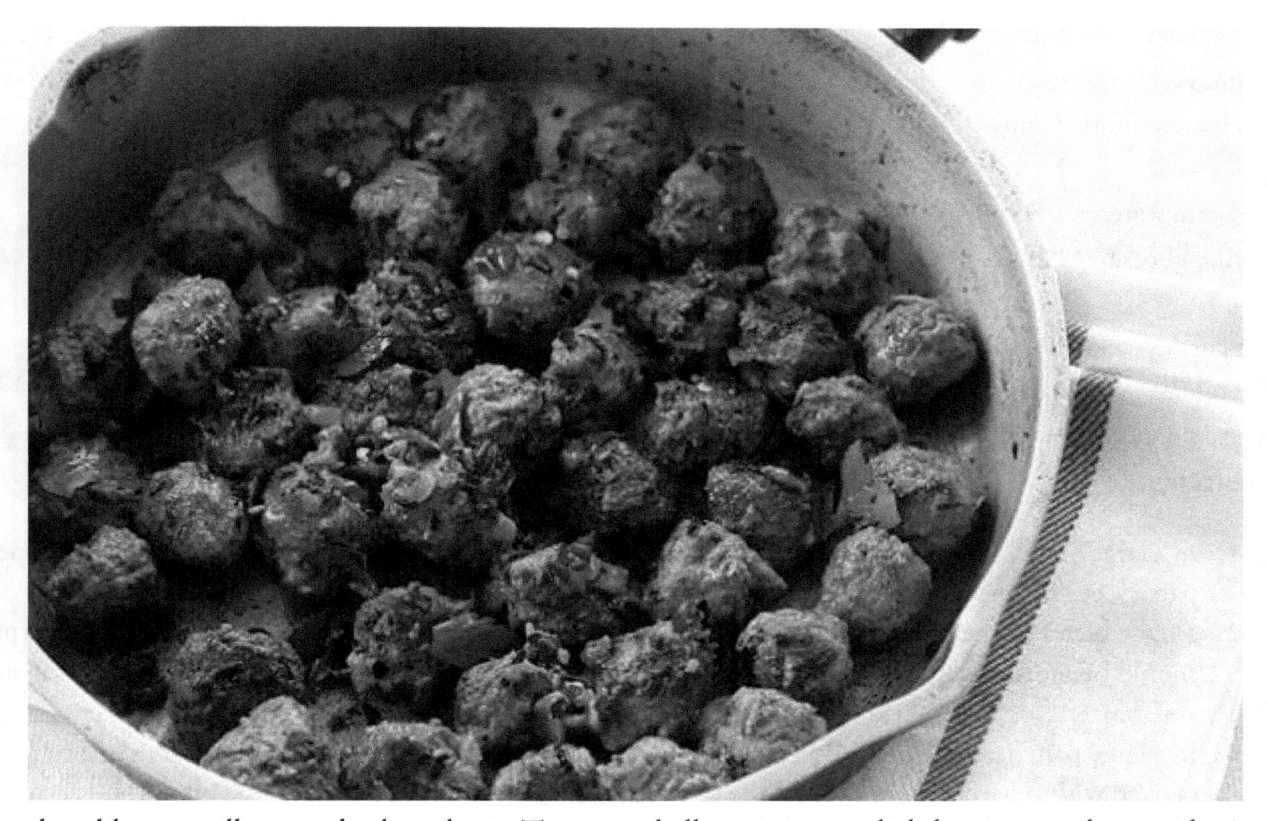

On the table, you will see an absolute classic. These meatballs are juicy yet slightly crispy on the outside. As you take a bite, the flavor is woeful and filling. This is perfectly accompanied by a fresh salad or on top of pasta.

Total: 50 minutes

Prep Time: 30 minutes

Cooking Time: 20 minutes

Serving Size: 8 servings

Ingredients	Measurements
Ground pork	½ lb
Ground beef	1 lb
Ground veal	½ lb
Fresh breadcrumbs	2 cups
Eggs	2
Lukewarm water	1 ½ cups
Pecorino cheese	1 cup
Garlic	2 cloves
Fresh parsley	1 ½ tbsp
Olive oil	1 cup
Salt and pepper	pinch

Directions:

1. In a large bowl, mix the ground meats with your hands until well combined. Then add in your chopped parsley, eggs, minced garlic, grated cheese, and some salt and pepper. Combine further.
2. Slowly blend in the breadcrumbs one cup at a time in combination with the water. The final texture should be moist and malleable, but not sticky. Use your palms to shape the meatballs to whatever size you desire.
3. In a large pan, heat up your olive oil and begin frying your meatballs in small batches until thoroughly cooked within with a slight char on the outside.
4. Drain the batches on paper towels and serve with whatever accompanying dish you have in mind.

Nifty Tips:

• It helps to cover your meatballs as they cook in olive oil so they retain their shape and don't become mushy.

• This is a base recipe for classic meatballs, and of course, you can zhuzh it up with hotter spices or different cheeses. The meatballs can be dropped in a pasta sauce, eaten with a fresh salad, or between two crispy pieces of bread.

• It is important to combine the different meats so as to create a flavorsome combination of fats and tastes. It does not necessarily need veal, but pork and beef are typical.

Chapter 14: Insalate [Salads]

Italians love their fresh and bitter salads. They also love bringing new and varied flavors from nuts, fruit, and diverse cheeses into a salad so that they transform something relatively boring into something amazing.

    I would like to show you a couple of recipes of fresh, gorgeously colorful, and brilliantly healthy salads that you will certainly appreciate. You can munch on these as a snack or as a side for any good meal. They are quick, easy, and innovative.

Orange and Fennel Salad

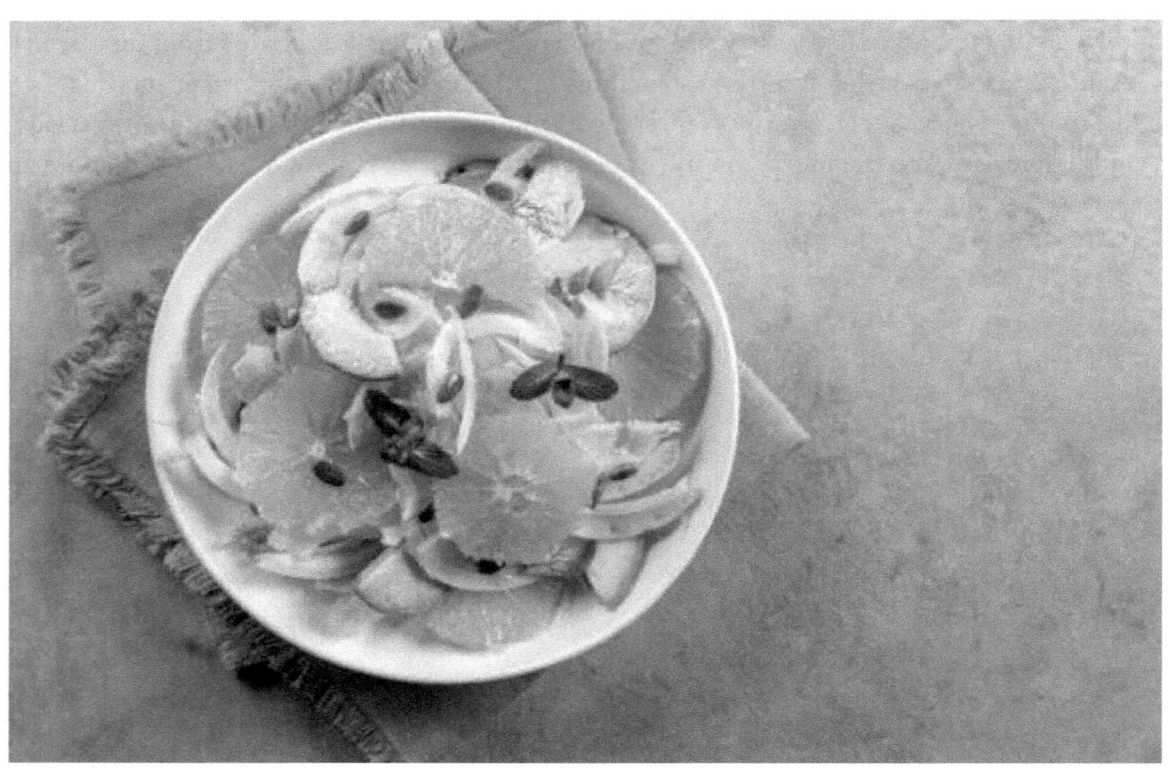

On the table you will see an immensely colorful and vibrant salad. Everything is on show, from the grilled chicken to the oranges and fennel. All these flavors might seem overpowering together, but when you taste it, you will realize how they balance so well, especially with the meaty kalamata olives!

Total Time: 20 minutes

Serving Size: 4 people

Ingredients	Measurements
Grilled chicken breasts	1 lb
Oranges	20 oz
Fennel	1 lb
Kalamata olives	½ cup
Rocket	10 oz
Sunflower seeds	¼ cup
Pistachios	¼ cup

Directions:

1. Take your grilled chicken breast and chop into bite-sized pieces.
2. To prepare the fennel, you need to chop off the core and stalks and then thinly slice.

3. Peel and wash your oranges, roughly chopping each slice.
4. Take your serving bowls and divide in the rocket; top with fennel, whole olives, seeds, and nuts. Finally, add in your chicken bits and garnish with your fennel fronds (leaves), then serve.

<u>Nifty Tips</u>:

- A great salad dressing for this is orange juice, olive oil, orange zest, and finely chopped garlic.

Caprese Salad

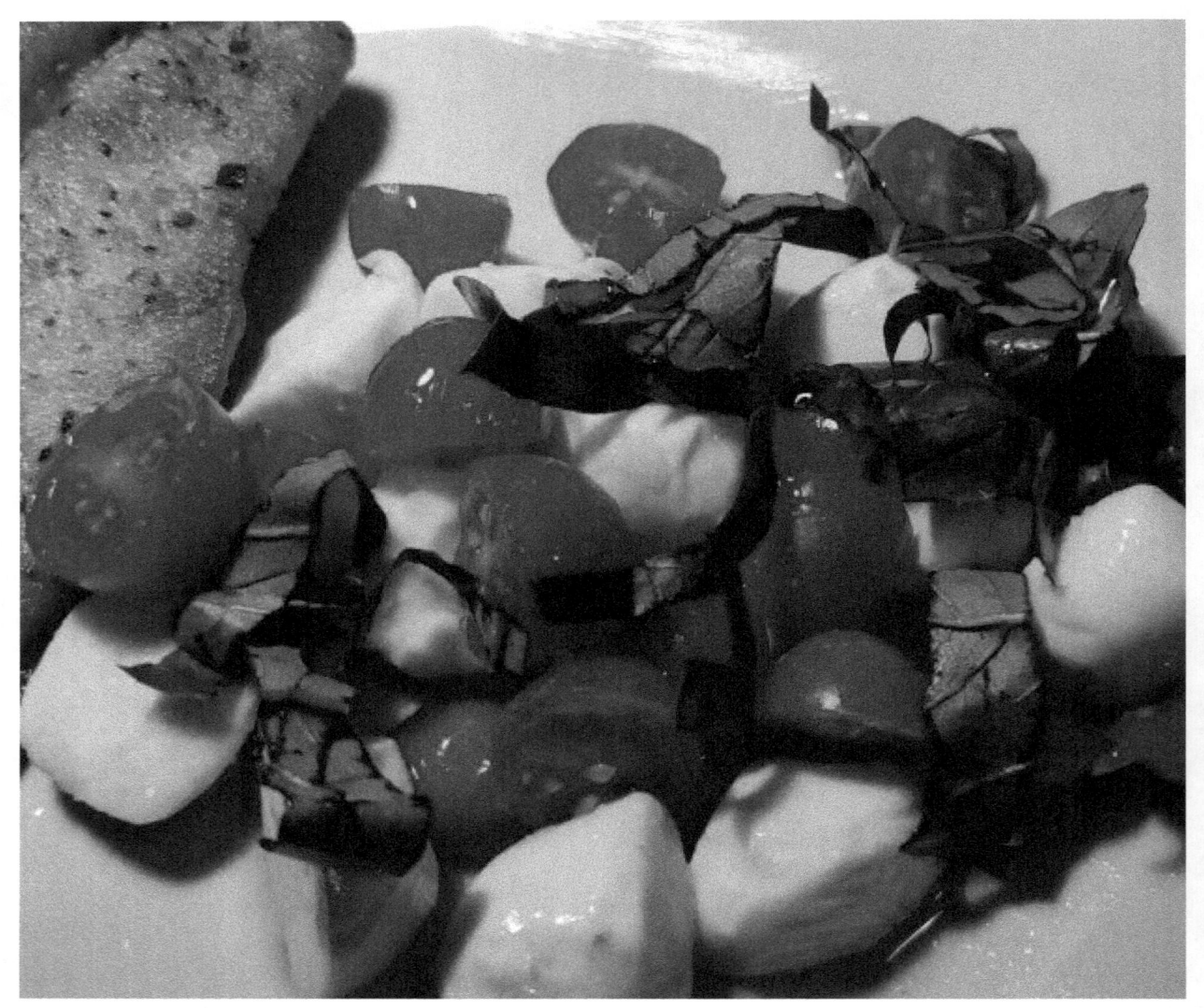

On the table you will see a classic salad that many people are very much aware of. The Caprese is a wonderful dish, so fresh and light, with ingredients that are wonderfully paired as well as being elegantly and effortlessly complementary.

<u>Total Time</u>: 25 minutes
<u>Serving Size</u>: 4 people

Ingredients	Measurements
Mozzarella	4 oz
Ripe tomatoes	1 lb
Fresh basil	handful
Olive oil	2 tbsp
Salt and pepper	Pinch

<u>Directions</u>:

1. Begin by slicing your tomatoes in irregular shapes, some sliced, some chopped.
2. Now we can tear the mozzarella cheese into small to medium chunks and do the same with the basil leaves, leaving some full.
3. Place the tomatoes and mozzarella onto the serving plate in a fishbone arrangement (layering), then drizzle with olive oil and sprinkle your salt and pepper.
4. Allow this to sit for 15 minutes so that the salt pulls from the tomatoes and leaves a juicy sauce for bread.

Chapter 15: Dolci [Desserts]

There is always space for dessert, right? Well, I always seem to find space, even after a big meal.

Italians love their desserts, and they will usually eat them accompanied by a post-dinner coffee or drink. It is a way to settle down after the exciting meal and conversation and before making your way to bed.

Wow! What a dinner we have had. Now to top it off with a final chapter on the sweeter things in life like semifreddo and tiramisú! These are classics each in their own right, and have a long-standing position as traditional, unchanged, and powerful desserts.

Honey Semifreddo

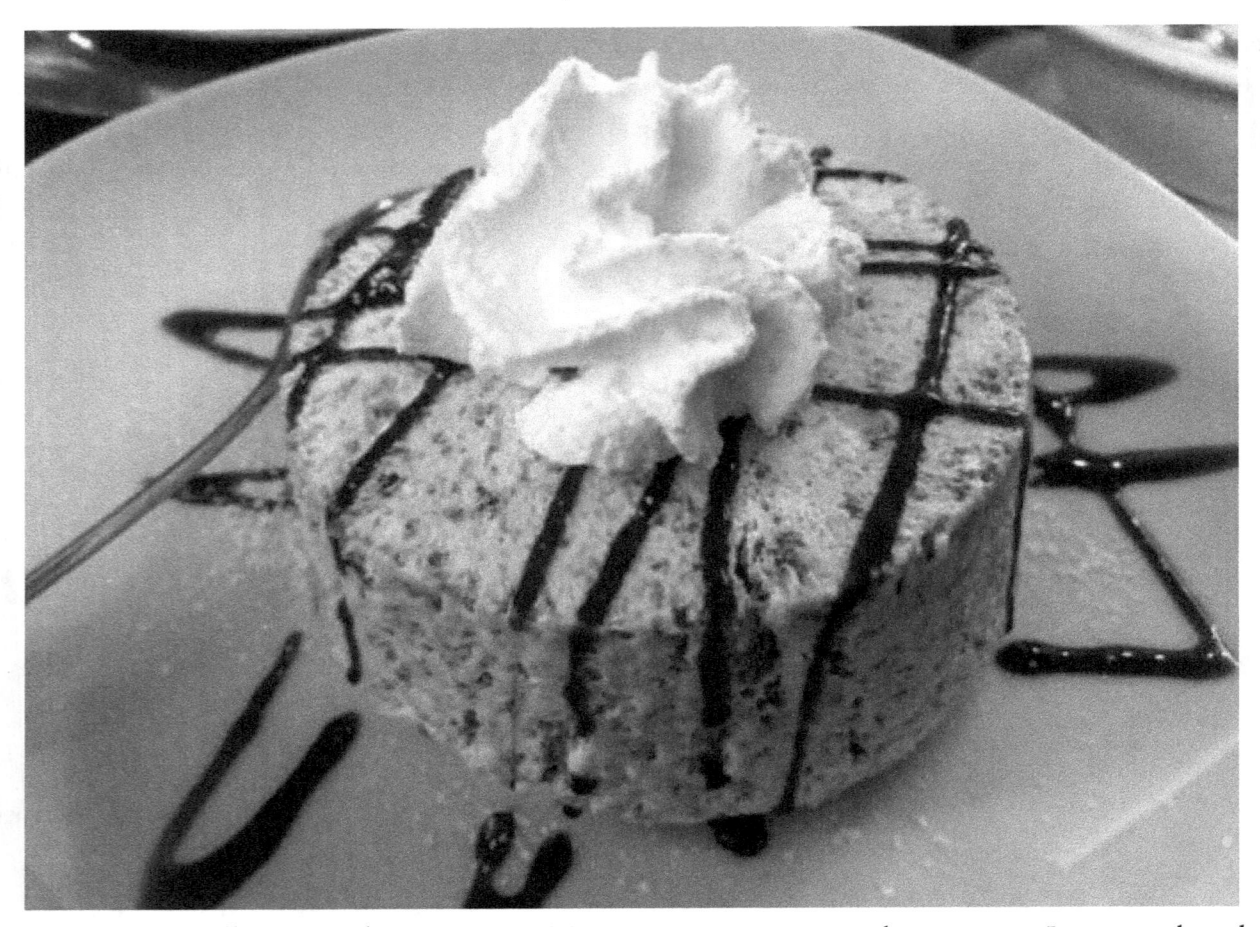

On the table you will see something gorgeous. This is not ice cream, or at least not yet. It is smooth and rich thanks to the honey and rosewater, but earthy and balanced thanks to the hint of salt, the nuts, and chocolate topping.

This dessert literally translates to "half cold," meaning that you can sit there guessing all day whether it's ice cream or not. Just don't miss out on the dessert! It will be gone in the blink of an eye.

<u>Total</u>: 8 hours 30 minutes
<u>Prep Time</u>: 8 hours (includes freezing time)
<u>Cooking Time</u>: 30 minutes
<u>Serving Size</u>: 8 servings

Ingredients	Measurements
Honey	¼ cup
Eggs	4 large
Rosewater	1 1/4 tsp
Heavy cream	8 oz
Vanilla extract	1 tsp
Shaved chocolate	Dressing
Toasted nuts	Dressing
Kosher salt	Pinch

<u>Special Equipment</u>:

- Food processor
- Loaf tin
- Dutch oven

- Food thermometer

<u>Directions</u>:

1. We begin by preparing the Dutch oven by filling ¼ with water, then placing in a crumpled ring of tinfoil at the base. This tin foil ring must sit above the waterline. Heat up your Dutch oven so the water begins to boil.
2. Line a loaf tin with plastic wrap so that it covers both the bottom and sides of the interior. Set aside.
3. Combine the heavy cream, rose water, and vanilla extract in the food processor at medium speed with a whisk attachment. Whisk until the mixture holds well to the beater when lifted.
4. Place the cream into a separate bowl and refrigerate till later.
5. Clean your stand mixer and place within it the eggs, honey, and salt, mixing until smooth.
6. Now, take care to place the mixing bowl into the Dutch oven so that it sits on top of the tinfoil, but does not touch the waterline. Allow this to steam for about 10 minutes, stirring continuously, adding in more boiling water as needed. The temperature needs to reach no more than 165 °F (74 °C), so keep an eye on the thermometer.
7. Next we will transfer the bowl back into the food processor with the same whisk attachment and whisk at a higher speed for 5 to 8 minutes until the eggs become foamy and get significantly larger in volume in a medium peak consistency.
8. Then remove the cream mixture from the fridge, and slowly add this into the egg mixture, half at a time. Once the mixture is smooth, fold it with a spatula until fully combined.
9. Now we can begin to insert the final mixture into the loaf tin, smooth out the surface, and place it in the freezer for 8 hours.
10. Once the dessert has set, you can free it from the tin using the plastic wrap to pull it out. Then you can

place it on a serving dish and return it to the freezer until ready to serve.
11. Chop up your toasted nuts and grab your shaved chocolate. Now you take your semifreddo out of the fridge and sprinkle on the toppings then serve immediately.

Nifty Tips:

- If you wish to have a smoother surface when serving, use baking paper, although it takes a little longer to prep.

- The tinfoil needs to be higher than the water level so that the mixing bowl does not touch the bottom of the Dutch oven or the water itself.

- If you are not using a food processor steel bowl, then make sure to use a glass mixing bowl as it creates a better steaming environment for the cream.

Tiramisú

On the table you will see a cake that is too beautiful for words. The creaminess of mascarpone, the richness yet subtle flavor of coffee, and the sweet biscuits within all play a symphony on your taste buds.

If you want a pick-me-up, then this cake is what you need. Don't be shy, indulge once in a while. It's good for you, and it's even better the next day.

<u>Total Time</u>: 8 hours 15 minutes (includes refrigeration time)

<u>Serving Size</u>: 8 servings

Ingredients	Measurements
Ladyfinger biscuits	24
Mascarpone	2 cups
Dark chocolate	3 tbsp
Strong brewed coffee	1 cup
Coffee liquor	4 tbsp
Cocoa powder	1 tbsp
Eggs	4
Sugar	6 tbsp

<u>Special Equipment</u>:

- Food processor

<u>Directions</u>:

1. First, we begin by placing two separate bowls in front of you. In each, place 3 tablespoons of sugar.
2. Next, you should be separating your eggs. In one bowl, we will place 4 egg yolks and in the other, 3 egg whites.
3. Whisk your egg whites and sugar by hand until nice and glossy. Then whisk your egg yolks and sugar in the food processor until well thickened.
4. In the egg yolk bowl, fold in your mascarpone until creamy and smooth.
5. Now we will fold ⅓ of the egg white mix into the mascarpone mix, slowly combining. Then you will proceed with the rest of the egg white mix until all is fully combined.
6. Make sure to have a medium to large ceramic or glass oven dish ready for the next step.
7. In a small shallow bowl pour in your coffee liquor and brewed coffee, and quickly dip each side of the ladyfingers into the coffee mix. Place the dipped lady fingers neatly at the base of the dish.
8. Next, we will layer half of the mascarpone mix over the soaked biscuits, spreading out evenly and topping with your grated dark chocolate. Repeat the process with another layer of biscuits and mascarpone, always topping with your remaining chocolate.
9. Sprinkle a touch of cocoa powder over the whole dessert and place it in the fridge for around 8 hours.

10. Serve when ready to have your dessert.

<u>Nifty Tips</u>:

- If your ladyfinger biscuits are too large for the dish, you can easily break them to fit.

- Always make sure to never contaminate the egg whites with the egg yolk or else the whisked mixture will collapse.

- You can easily swap out the coffee liquor for an amaretto or any other thick Italian liquor.

- Try using proper Italian Savoiardi biscuits that hold their shape and texture.

Conclusion

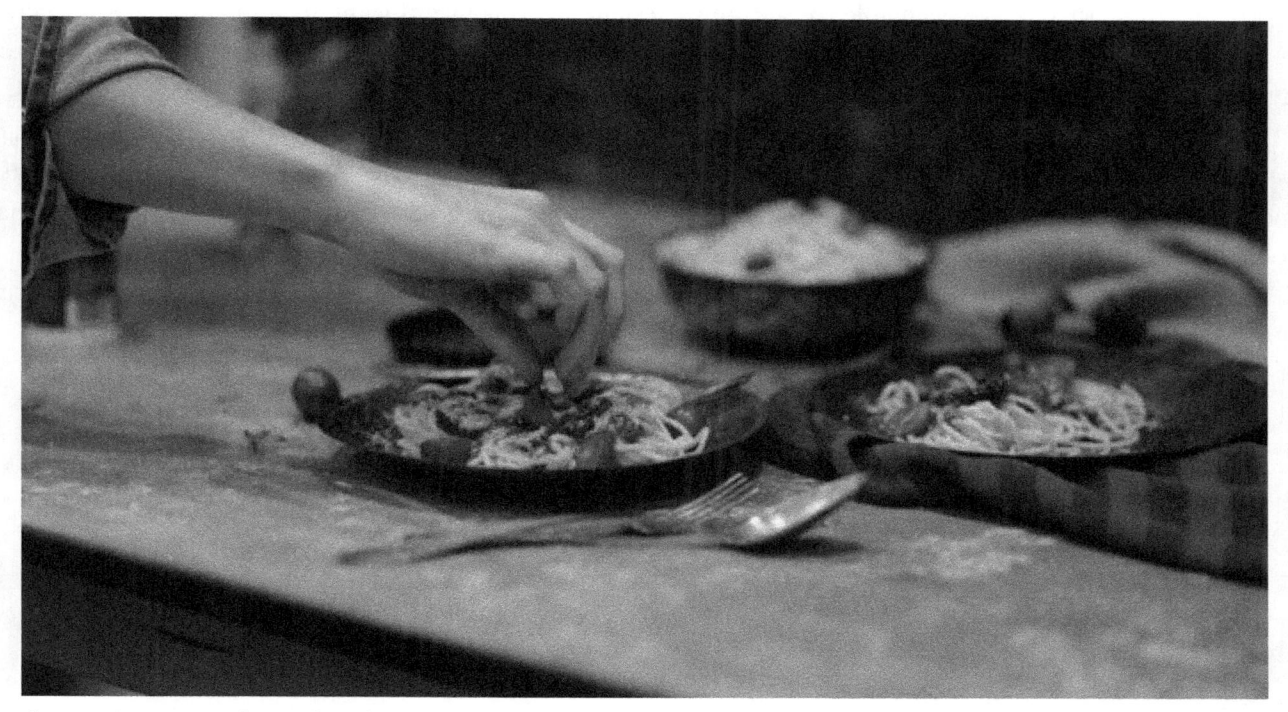

You know this is not the end, right?

This is just the beginning of your journey into the marvels of Italian cooking and because you have just dipped your toes into the beauty of the cuisine, you are now more curious than before.

Remember, you have been more than courageous in your pursuit, you have been respectful! Finding keen interest in the culture and the tradition is how you honor the cuisine.

Of course, I must thank you for taking up the opportunity to learn more about the most loved food in the world. Not only are you bettering yourself everyday with your interest, but you are also showing others how easy it is to grow in a culinary art.

By reviewing the history of the cuisine, we were able to assess that what we know as Italian food today is a very complex and inspiring story of a country. Italy and its cuisine are inexplicably interconnected both in tragedy and joy, poverty and wealth, tradition and modern influence.

Then we started looking deeper into what the cuisine itself stands for. Finding that its popularity stems from its subtle statement of simplicity and taste. We broke down the aspects of the cuisine into its core foundations and explored the idea of cooking like a real Italian mamma. We would not have gotten very far without having jumped into the basic ingredients that you would find in a kitchen and what role they each play in the bigger picture. And of course, the 50 recipes that I have lovingly shared with you, each with distinct and interesting flavors that are never really set in stone, can be a guide to allow you to become more creative. If the mood strikes, these recipes can be altered, molded, and envisioned differently depending on your preference.

With such a vast variety of delicious and easy to prepare recipes, I really believe that you're all set to entertain your taste buds and impress your family and guests with these delectable Italian recipes.

I truly hope that I have been able to capture the essence of this magnificent art and allowed you to come to the realization that the real chemistry here is in the joy you have when you boil your pasta, chop your fresh herbs, sear your meat, and bring it all together at the end for a finale.

While I enjoy bringing easy food to everyone's home, writing a book about recipes is never an easy job, especially while keeping up with my full time job as a chef. But hey! This is what I live for, and this is what makes me feel alive! I do it with a smile and a hope that it has made your life a whole lot more exciting and passionate too.

Of course, this book will not be my last, so by leaving a quick 2 minute review, it can go a long way in supporting me towards creating more recipe books that you can enjoy from the comfort of your home.

Thank you once again. And may your journey in the discovery of gastronomy never cease.

Quick Conversion Charts

Weight

Pounds (lb)	Ounces (oz)	Grams (gr)
¼	4	125
½	8	250
1	16	500
1 ½	24	750
2	32	1 kg
3	48	1.5 kg

Volume

Tablespoon (Tbsp)	Cups	Ounces (Oz)	Milliliter (ml)
1		½	15
2		1	30
3		1 ½	45
4	¼	2	60
6	⅓	3	90
8	½	4	125
	1	8	250
	2	16	500
	4	32	1 liter

Oven Temperatures Rule

F° → C°: (F°-32) x 5/9 [minus 32, multiple that by 5 and then divide by 9]
C° → F°: (C°x 9/5) + 32 [multiply by 9, divide by 5, and add 32]

References

Achitoff-Gray, N. (2020, September 3). *Salumi 101: your guide to Italy's finest cured meats*. Serious Eats. https://www.seriouseats.com/salumi-guide-italian-cured-meats-salami-prosciutto

Achitoff-Gray, N. (2021, March 7). *The science of the best fresh pasta*. Serious Eats. https://www.seriouseats.com/best-easy-all-purpose-fresh-pasta-dough-recipe-instructions

Alfaro, D. (2019, September 17). *Basic culinary arts knife cuts and shapes*. The Spruce Eats. https://www.thespruceeats.com/culinary-arts-knife-cuts-photo-gallery-4121795

Allrecipes. (2013, October 20). *How to make homemade pasta*. Allrecipes. https://www.youtube.com/watch?v=03foJzD64DA

Babish Culinary Universe. (2017, November 17). *Pasta - Basics with Babish*. Www.youtube.com. https://www.youtube.com/watch?v=HdSLKZ6LN94

Basics of baking bread. (2020, January 22). *The basics of bread. An Italian bread recipe*. The Redhead Baker. https://www.theredheadbaker.com/basics-of-baking-bread-italian-bread-recipe/

Bezzone, F. (2019a, September 3). *History of Italian Renaissance cuisine and the Middle Ages*. Life in Italy. https://lifeinitaly.com/the-history-of-italian-cuisine-ii/

Bezzone, F. (2019b, September 11). *History of Italian cuisine in the 17th, 18th, and 19th centuries*. Life in Italy. https://lifeinitaly.com/the-history-of-italian-cuisine-iii/

Bezzone, F. (2019c, October 5). *History of Italian cuisine in the 20th century*. Life in Italy. https://lifeinitaly.com/history-italian-cuisine-iv/

Bezzone, F. (2019d, October 30). *The history of Italian cuisine I*. Life in Italy. https://lifeinitaly.com/the-history-of-italian-cuisine-i/

Calzone with ricotta. (2019, July 23). *Calzone with ricotta & prosciutto*. Eataly. https://www.eataly.com/us_en/magazine/eataly-recipes/calzone-recipe-ricotta-prosciutto/

Chef Studio. (2020, March 21). *How to make pasta without a machine*. Www.youtube.com; Chef Studio. https://www.youtube.com/watch?v=UfvrcHzv4TQ

Christensen, E. (2013, August 21). *How to make homemade ricotta cheese*. Kitchn; Apartment Therapy, LLC. https://www.thekitchn.com/how-to-make-homemade-ricotta-cheese-cooking-lessons-from-the-kitchn-23326

D'Acampo, G. (2018, October 18). *Sautéed prawns with garlic and chili.* Gino D'Acampo. https://ginodacampo.com/courses/antipasti-recipes/

D'Acampo, G. (2019, October 31). *Genovese mussels with pesto and olives.* Gino D'Acampo. https://ginodacampo.com/courses/antipasti-recipes/

Del Conte, A. (2016, May 16). *Ten commandments of Italian cooking.* The Guardian. https://www.theguardian.com/lifeandstyle/2016/may/16/ten-commandments-of-italian-cooking

El-Waylly, S. (2020, March 19). *Pressure cooker corn risotto recipe.* Serious Eats. https://www.seriouseats.com/pressure-cooker-corn-risotto

Essential pantry staples. (2021, March 17). *Essential pantry staples for better pasta.* Serious Eats. https://www.seriouseats.com/pasta-pantry-staples

Fincher, M. (2021, April 14). *27 types of pasta and their uses.* Allrecipes. https://www.allrecipes.com/article/types-of-pasta/

Flay, B. (2015, September 4). *Pizza dough.* Foodnetwork.com. https://www.foodnetwork.com/recipes/bobby-flay/pizza-dough-recipe-1921714

Fried baby artichokes. (2007, January). *Fried baby artichokes recipe.* Food & Wine. https://www.foodandwine.com/recipes/fried-baby-artichokes

Gauchat, S., & Gold, B. (2012, March 9). *An introduction to Italian cuisine.* Real Simple; Real Simple. https://www.realsimple.com/food-recipes/cooking-tips-techniques/italian-cuisine

Gavin, J. (2020, July 27). *Bruschetta with tomato and basil.* Jessica Gavin Culinary Scientist. https://www.jessicagavin.com/classic-italian-bruschetta/

Gore, M. (2021, June 25). *Slow-cooker chicken cacciatore.* Easy dinner win. Delish. https://www.delish.com/cooking/recipe-ideas/a23106011/slow-cooker-chicken-cacciatore-recipe/

Grilled zucchini. (2013, August). *Grilled zucchini with fresh mozzarella recipe.* Food & Wine. https://www.foodandwine.com/recipes/grilled-zucchini-fresh-mozzarella

Gritzer, D. (2018, August 29). *Veneto-style radicchio risotto with walnuts and blue cheese recipe.* Serious Eats. https://www.seriouseats.com/radicchio-risotto-blue-cheese-walnuts-thyme-veneto-recipe

Gritzer, D. (2019a, February 5). *Osso buco (Italian braised veal shanks) recipe.* Serious Eats. https://www.seriouseats.com/osso-buco-italian-braised-veal-shanks-recipe

Gritzer, D. (2019b, May 8). *How to cook Italian food like an Italian*. Serious Eats. https://www.seriouseats.com/the-essential-steps-to-mastering-italian-cuisine

Gritzer, D. (2021a, March 7). *How salty should pasta water be?* Serious Eats. https://www.seriouseats.com/how-salty-should-pasta-water-be

Gritzer, D. (2021b, March 7). *Pasta ai quattro formaggi (creamy four-cheese pasta) recipe*. Serious Eats. https://www.seriouseats.com/pasta-ai-quattro-formaggi

Gritzer, D. (2021c, March 7). *Roman-style spaghetti alla carrettiera (tomato, tuna, and mushroom pasta) recipe*. Serious Eats. https://www.seriouseats.com/roman-style-spaghetti-alla-carrettiera-tomato-tuna-and-mushroom-pasta

Gritzer, D. (2021d, March 12). *Basic ragù bolognese recipe*. Serious Eats. https://www.seriouseats.com/basic-ragu-bolognese-recipe

Gritzer, D. (2021e, March 12). *Spaghetti aglio e olio (pasta in garlic and oil sauce) recipe*. Serious Eats. https://www.seriouseats.com/spaghetti-aglio-olio-recipe

Gritzer, D. (2021f, April 26). *Smooth and creamy polenta recipe*. Serious Eats. https://www.seriouseats.com/smooth-creamy-polenta-recipe

Gritzer, D. (2021g, December 15). *How to roast a whole fish in a salt crust*. Serious Eats. https://www.seriouseats.com/salt-baked-whole-fish-with-fresh-herbs-5212108

Heeley, B. (2021, April 9). *Eating like an Italian: food norms, beliefs, and etiquette*. Welcome to Italy. https://romancandletours.com/blog/2018/10/12/eating-like-an-italian-food-norms-beliefs-and-etiquette/

Italian cuisine keeps spreading. (2019, April 29). *How Italian cuisine keeps spreading all over the globe*. Travel with Pedro. https://www.travelwithpedro.com/how-italian-cuisine-keeps-spreading-all-over-the-globe/

Italian cuisine popularity. (2021, August 15). *Why is Italian cuisine so popular around the world?* Italian Street Kitchen Australia. https://italianstreetkitchen.com/au/news/why-is-italian-cuisine-so-popular-around-the-world/

Italian terms. (2018, September 28). *Italian food and cooking terms and glossary*. Www.gayot.com. https://www.gayot.com/food-cooking/italian-food-terms/

Kemp, E. (2017, December 29). *Easy marinated olives - Ready in 5 minutes*. Inside the Rustic Kitchen. https://www.insidetherustickitchen.com/easy-marinated-olives/

Kemp, E. (2018, October 6). *Fried sage leaves with anchovies*. Inside the Rustic Kitchen. https://www.insidetherustickitchen.com/fried-sage-anchovies/

Kemp, E. (2019, November 16). *Sausage stuffed mushrooms with gorgonzola*. Inside the Rustic Kitchen. https://www.insidetherustickitchen.com/sausage-stuffed-mushrooms-gorgonzola-walnuts/

Kemp, E. (2020a, July 28). *Whipped ricotta dip with roasted tomatoes*. Inside the Rustic Kitchen. https://www.insidetherustickitchen.com/whipped-ricotta-dip-roasted-tomatoes/

Kemp, E. (2020b, July 30). *Fried zucchini pizza bites*. Inside the Rustic Kitchen. https://www.insidetherustickitchen.com/fried-zucchini-pizza-bites/

Kemp, E. (2020c, September 8). *Grissini - Italian breadsticks*. Inside the Rustic Kitchen. https://www.insidetherustickitchen.com/grissini/

Kemp, E. (2021a, April 6). *Torta pasqualina (spinach & ricotta egg pie)*. Inside the Rustic Kitchen. https://www.insidetherustickitchen.com/torta-pasqualina/

Kemp, E. (2021b, April 29). *Baked ricotta with thyme and parmesan*. Inside the Rustic Kitchen. https://www.insidetherustickitchen.com/baked-ricotta/

Kemp, E. (2021c, November 29). *Mozzarella bocconcini, pesto and sun blushed tomatoes*. Inside the Rustic Kitchen. https://www.insidetherustickitchen.com/mozzarella-bocconcini/

Kemp, E. (2021d, December 1). *Walnut focaccia*. Inside the Rustic Kitchen. https://www.insidetherustickitchen.com/walnut-focaccia/

Lentil soup. (2016, January 8). *Italian lentil soup*. Gimme Some Oven. https://www.gimmesomeoven.com/italian-lentil-soup-recipe/

López-Alt, J. K. (2019, March 21). *Quick and easy homemade ricotta gnocchi recipe*. Serious Eats. https://www.seriouseats.com/ricotta-gnocchi-homemade-food-lab-recipe

López-Alt, J. K. (2020a, March 21). *Perfect risotto recipe*. Serious Eats. https://www.seriouseats.com/how-to-make-perfect-risotto-recipe

López-Alt, J. K. (2020b, September 9). *How to chop capers and olives*. Knife Skills. Serious Eats. https://www.seriouseats.com/knife-skills-how-to-chop-capers-and-olives

López-Alt, J. K. (2021a, March 7). *The right way to sauce pasta*. Serious Eats. https://www.seriouseats.com/the-right-way-to-sauce-pasta

López-Alt, J. K. (2021b, March 12). *Pasta alla norma (Sicilian pasta with eggplant, tomatoes, and ricotta salata).* Serious Eats. https://www.seriouseats.com/sicilian-style-pasta-with-eggplant-tomatoes-ricotta-salata-pasta-alla-norma-recipe

López-Alt, J. K. (2021c, March 17). *Spaghetti puttanesca (spaghetti with capers, olives, and anchovies).* Serious Eats. https://www.seriouseats.com/spaghetti-puttanesca-pasta-week-capers-olives-anchovies-recipe

López-Alt, J. K. (2021d, April 7). *Ricotta gnocchi with asparagus and prosciutto recipe.* Serious Eats. https://www.seriouseats.com/ricotta-gnocchi-asparagus-prosciutto

López-Alt, J. K. (2022, February 14). *The best Italian-American tomato sauce recipe.* Serious Eats. https://www.seriouseats.com/the-best-slow-cooked-italian-american-tomato-sauce-red-sauce-recipe

Marshall, C. (2021, September 23). *21 classic Italian soup recipes.* The Kitchen Community. https://thekitchencommunity.org/italian-soup-recipes/

Marx, S. (2020, May 5). *No-knead skillet focaccia is a faster way to flavorful, homemade bread.* Serious Eats. https://www.seriouseats.com/easy-no-knead-focaccia

Marx, S. (2021a, March 22). *Creamy pasta with mushrooms.* Serious Eats. https://www.seriouseats.com/mushroom-pasta-creamy

Marx, S. (2021b, December 15). *Fritto misto di mare (fried mixed seafood).* Serious Eats. https://www.seriouseats.com/fritto-misto-di-mare-fried-mixed-seafood-5212686

Marx, S. (2021c, December 15). *Risotto ai gamberi (shrimp risotto).* Serious Eats. https://www.seriouseats.com/risotto-con-i-gamberi-risotto-with-shrimp-5212626

Mckenney, S. (2016, July 12). *Zucchini & herbed ricotta flatbread.* Sally's Baking Addiction. https://sallysbakingaddiction.com/zucchini-herbed-ricotta-flatbread/

Meatballs. (2022). *The best meatballs.* Allrecipes. https://www.allrecipes.com/recipe/40399/the-best-meatballs/

Mele, D. (2008, May 28). *Basic Italian bread.* Italian Food Forever. https://www.italianfoodforever.com/2008/05/basic-italian-bread-2/

Mele, D. (2020, September 29). *Italian easy: risotto with spring peas, ham, and Fontina.* Serious Eats. https://www.seriouseats.com/everday-italian-risotto-with-spring-peas-ham

Orange and fennel salad. (2020, August 17). *Insalata di arance e finocchi (orange and fennel salad)*. Summer Yule Nutrition. https://summeryule.com/insalata-di-arance-e-finocchi-orange-and-fennel-salad/

Overhiser, S. (2020, April 23). *Pasta e ceci (Italian chickpea soup)*. A Couple Cooks. https://www.acouplecooks.com/pasta-e-ceci-italian-chickpea-soup/

Parisi, B. (2019, November 7). *Zuppa Toscana soup recipe*. Chef Billy Parisi. https://www.billy-parisi.com/zuppa-toscana-soup-recipe/

Piran, N. (2016, October 23). *Sausage arugula pizza*. The Bitter Side of Sweet. https://www.thebittersideofsweet.com/sausage-arugula-pizza/

Polenta concia. (2019). *Polenta concia*. Great Italian Chefs. https://www.greatitalianchefs.com/recipes/polenta-concia-recipe

Prior, E. (2020, July 3). *21 different types of Italian breads*. Flavours Holidays. https://www.flavoursholidays.co.uk/blog/21-types-italian-breads/

Scarpaleggia, G. (2015, November 26). *The foundations of Italian cooking*. Great Italian Chefs. https://www.greatitalianchefs.com/features/odori-battuto-soffritto

Segal, J. (2019, October 31). *Italian wedding soup*. Once upon a Chef. https://www.onceuponachef.com/recipes/italian-wedding-soup.html

Sert, A. N. (2017). *Italian cuisine: characteristics and effects*. Journal of Business Management and Economic Research, 1(1), 49–57. https://doi.org/10.29226/jobmer.2017.4

Smith, M. (2019, March 12). *Italian cuisine is world's most popular*. Yougov.co.uk. https://yougov.co.uk/topics/food/articles-reports/2019/03/12/italian-cuisine-worlds-most-popular

Soranidis, A. (2019, November 6). *Authentic Italian potato frittata*. The Petite Cook^{TM}. https://www.thepetitecook.com/italian-potato-frittata/

Top Italian cheeses. (2021, August 27). *Top cheeses loved and used by Italians*. Rifugios - Country Italian Cuisine. https://www.ilcafferifugio.com/top-italian-cheeses-loved-and-used-by-many/

Tuscan steak. (2022). *Tuscan flank steak*. Allrecipes. https://www.allrecipes.com/recipe/229452/tuscan-flank-steak/

Why Italian food is so popular. (2020, July 29). *4 reasons why Italian food is so popular*. Chef Gourmet LLC. https://chefgourmetllc.com/reasons-why-italian-food-is-popular/

Yetter, E. (2021, October 12). *Easy Italian bread*. The Spruce Eats. https://www.thespruceeats.com/italian-bread-428161

Zehr, D. (2015, May 15). *Pizza margherita, fast and easy - Only 20 minutes from prep to first bite!* Parade: Entertainment, Recipes, Health, Life, Holidays. https://parade.com/841371/danzehr/pizza-margherita-fast-and-easy-only-20-minutes-from-prep-to-first-bite/

Zuppa Toscana. (2022). *Super delicious zuppa Toscana*. Allrecipes. https://www.allrecipes.com/recipe/143069/super-delicious-zuppa-toscana/

Image References

Aedrozda (2015, November 18). [Arugula pizza]. https://pixabay.com/photos/pizza-food-healthy-kitchen-lunch-1047391/

Adom, R. (2020, December 15). [Marinated olives and grissini]. https://pixabay.com/photos/grapes-breadstick-olives-nuts-food-5829405/

Alexanrove, V. (2019, September 16). [tiramisu] https://unsplash.com/photos/0DIJIynObx4

Anshu, A. (2020, April 26). [Frittata]. https://unsplash.com/photos/wmmLnCBcD-o

Claire, R. (2020, November 12). [Meatballs]. https://www.pexels.com/photo/red-tomatoes-beside-a-sliced-bread-5863610/

Deaner, D. (2019, May 3). [Kitchen tools]. https://unsplash.com/photos/d9qnD33cBJs

De la Marza, I. (2020, November 15). [Focaccia]. https://unsplash.com/photos/s2VbmuZzo60

Deluvio, C. (2020, March 31). [Creamy mushroom pasta]. https://unsplash.com/photos/vUE2mIFb8lE

Du Preez, P. (2018, June 10). *People eating a meal around the table*. https://unsplash.com/photos/W3SEyZODn8U

Gumenuiek, A. (2020, May 19). [Cheese platter]. https://unsplash.com/photos/_wdXUGB2GO4

Kapusnak, J. (2017, June 27). *Colorful Italian ingredients*. https://unsplash.com/photos/tEVisOXz26Y

Rita, E. (2017, July 24). [Osso buco]. https://pixabay.com/photos/ossobuco-flesh-calf-veal-beef-2535546/

Rita, E. (2020, July 7). [Semifreddo]. https://pixabay.com/photos/parfait-semifreddo-cold-cream-5377688/

Rithwick. (2018, January 15). *Food photography*. https://unsplash.com/photos/SpXtY0d7VF0

Spetnitskaya, N. (2018, February 3). *Dough and hands*. https://unsplash.com/photos/tOYiQxF9-Ys

Thorsten, F. (2019, June 19). [Classic bruschetta]. https://pixabay.com/photos/bruschetta-tomatoes-food-loaf-4282898/

Travels, F. (2018, August 19). *Italian pizza and wine.* https://unsplash.com/photos/W01Qwuhb_l4

Tripkovic, K. (2018, March 22). [Cutting pasta]. https://unsplash.com/photos/EGmwwDzme6s

Tumanyan, K. (2020, April 6). *Lasagna recipe.* https://unsplash.com/photos/lXTOsdII3DE

Zapata, J. (2015, November 12). *Making Pasta.* https://unsplash.com/photos/4nXkhLCrkLo

Don't miss out!

Visit the website below and you can sign up to receive emails whenever Maleb Braine publishes a new book. There's no charge and no obligation.

https://books2read.com/r/B-A-WOXU-CFABC

BOOKS2READ

Connecting independent readers to independent writers.

Also by Maleb Braine

Everyday cookbook series.
French cookbook for everyday use.
Italian Cookbook for everyday use.
Bread baking cookbook you need every day
A baking cookbook you need Every Day

CPSIA information can be obtained
at www.ICGtesting.com
Printed in the USA
BVHW012012221022
649988BV00017B/11